THE GOLD'S GYM

BOOK OF
STRENGTH TRAINING
FOR ATHLETES

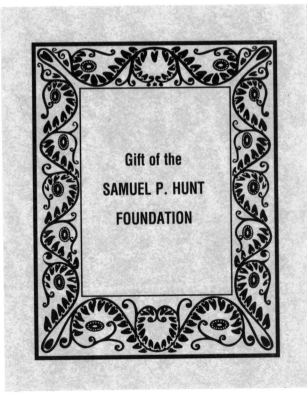

Other books by Ken Sprague
Sports Strength
The Athlete's Body
The Gold's Gym Book of Bodybuilding
The Gold's Gym Book of Weight Training
Weight and Strength Training for Kids and Teenagers

THE
GOLD'S GYM
BOOK OF
STRENGTH TRAINING
FOR ATHLETES

Ken Sprague

Photography by John Bauguess

A Perigee Book

This book, with my warmest regards, is dedicated to Ken Waller,
Dan Howard, Kent Kuehn, and Bill Reynolds—four guys who never
received the credit they deserved for the success of Gold's Gym.

Perigee Books
are published by
The Berkley Publishing Group
200 Madison Avenue
New York, NY 10016

Library of Congress Cataloging-in-Publication Data

♯ 29389160

Sprague, Ken.
   The Gold's Gym book of strength training for athletes/by Ken
Sprague; photography by John Baugess.
      p.   cm.
   "A Perigee book."
   ISBN 0-399-51863-0
   1. Weight training.   2. Exercise.   3. Muscle strength.   I. Title.
II. Title: Book of strength training for athletes.
GV546.S69   1994   93-45040 CIP
613.7'13—dc20

Cover design © 1994 by Andrew M. Newman
Cover photo © 1993 by Soloflex, Inc.
Printed in the United States of America
1 2 3 4 5 6 7 8 9 10

This book is printed on acid-free paper.
                    ∞

The strength-training routines in this book are intended
for healthy individuals. People with health problems
should not follow these routines without a physician's
approval. Before beginning any exercise or nutrition
program, always consult with your doctor. Children should
always be supervised by an adult while performing these
exercises.

CONTENTS

Acknowledgments

• Thank you, Jeremy Tarcher, for your efforts toward the first edition of this book.
• Thank you, Donna Wong, a wonderful wife, for your unwavering support and tireless efforts in pulling this edition together.
• Thank you, Laura Shepherd and Lisa Swayne, for your editorial assistance.
• Thank you, John Bauguess and Ron Finne, for the fine photography in this book.
• Thank you, Molly Beauchamp, Bruce Budzig, Owen Englemann, Mike Estes, Robert Hausmann, Aubree Knecht, Sheila Kryl, Robin Mitzel, Ember Parks, Matt Powers, Gina Simontacchi, Chris Sprague, Greg Thompson, and Jacque Till for making this a better-looking book.
• Thank you, Brian Romine and Mark Delp, for your advice.
• Thank you to the following equipment companies for contributing photographs and information to update this book: Cybex®, Soloflex®, Nautilus®, Nordic Flex Gold®, Speed City, Stair-Master®, Universal®, and Vasa.

Preface

The Gold's Gym Book of Strength Training for Athletes provides you with a proven, nuts-and-bolts, no-nonsense approach to strength training that will help you build a stronger, quicker, more athletic body.

Why and how *you* should train are detailed throughout the book. You must supply the training effort. There is nothing too intellectual to inhibit your strength gains, because strength training needn't be an intellectual pursuit. On the other hand, there is nothing physically easy included here, because strength training requires physical exertion. But if you supply the effort to succeed, *The Gold's Gym Book of Strength Training for Athletes* is your bridge to success.

If you're new to strength training, reading the book from cover to cover offers a complete strength-training course. The early chapters provide you with the basic training information and physiological concepts you'll need in order to appreciate the rationale for the strength-training workouts detailed in later chapters.

If you are an advanced strength trainer, I suggest that you use chapters 1 through 6 as continuing resource material. Chapters 7 through 10 offer guidelines for more sophisticated, personalized strength-training workouts to better meet the strength demands of your specific sport.

What you won't find in the book are promises of quick fixes, because successful strength training requires continuing commitment. The average NFL football player has been strength training for 6 years before entering the league. Every modern decathlon champion has been a longtime strength trainer before winning a gold medal. All major league baseball teams have strength programs. The best tennis players, boxers, and rowers strength train throughout their careers. Strength training works—if the athlete is committed to making it work. And it works equally well for professionals, high school athletes, and weekend basketball players.

Whether the arena is a high school gymnasium or an Olympic stadium, all athletes dream of running a little faster, jumping a little higher, or throwing a little farther. *The Gold's Gym Book of Strength Training for Athletes* offers the chance to make those dreams come true.

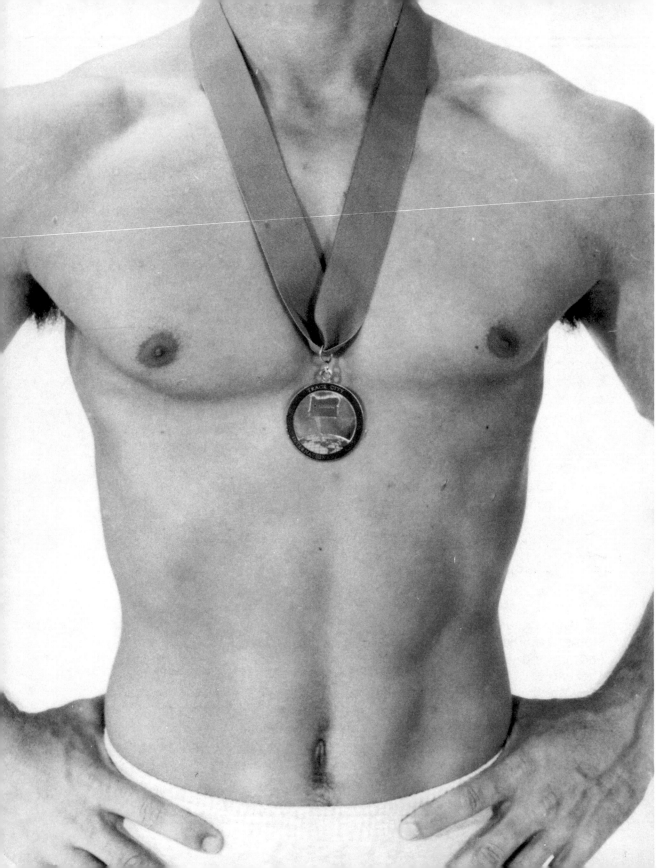

1
WHY STRENGTH TRAIN?

At some point in the career of every serious athlete comes the decision to strength train. They strength train to become the best they can be, knowing that every jump, swing, stride, or throw improves with the strength of his or her muscles.

Bodybuilding and Strength Training:
Very Different Goals

Both use much the same equipment, but strength training and bodybuilding have very different goals and training programs. The most obvious are:

- The goal of strength training is stronger muscles and movements;
- The goal of bodybuilding is a change in physical appearance;
- Strength training programs differ from bodybuilding programs in the number of sets and reps, training frequency, exercise selection, and intensity.

Regardless of the sport, strength training provides a competitive edge. Given identical twins, and all other factors being equal, the stronger twin will run and swim faster, hit a ball farther, and jump higher. In short, a stronger athlete is a better athlete. That's why so many athletes have climbed aboard the strength training bandwagon.

Competitions are won and lost on the practice field is a coaching axiom that reflects the importance of maximizing your training time. In fact, maximizing your training time is the greatest hurdle that you'll encounter during your athletic career.

Over the past 25 years, Gold's Gym has helped thousands of men and women to maximize their training time and become better athletes. Both professional and amateur athletes—as well as individuals from such diverse walks of life as medicine, business, and education—have come to the most famous weight-training gym in the world to train with the best.

While Gold's has gained an international reputation as the gym where famous bodybuilders like Lou Ferrigno and Arnold Schwarzenegger have trained, a far greater percentage of the gym's members are high school, college, and professional athletes seeking a higher level of performance. But it isn't necessary to train at a Gold's Gym to benefit from strength training, because with this book you can turn any weight room—garage, basement, school gym, or another commercial gymnasium—into a successful training center.

Where you train is far less important than *how* you train. In this book you will learn the proven methods of strength training that can be applied to any gym in the country. Every exercise, every training technique, and every workout has endured countless practical tests and proven to be effective in elevating individual sports performance. If you follow the recommended procedures in this book, you too will increase your athletic performance.

STRENGTH TRAINING AND SPORTS PERFORMANCE

Strength is only one component of athletic ability. Speed, endurance, reaction time, psychological preparedness, flexibility, and technique count too. But of all the components that mesh into a complete athletic performance, strength is the easiest and the quickest to improve.

Strength training involves pushing, pulling, or twisting against resistance; that resistance is usually a barbell or machine. Over time, pushing or pulling against resistance gradually strengthens your *skeletal muscles.*

Skeletal muscles are the muscles of sport. They're the muscles that attach to a pair of bones, moving the body as they contract. They are the muscles responsible for bending the elbows, straightening the legs, grasping a barbell, and all other athletic movements. The synchronous contractions of many skeletal muscles are the agents of the multiple movements of your athletic event. The stronger the muscles, the greater force and efficiency of those movements.

Strength training takes many forms, such as exercising with weights attached to your ankles, wrists, or waist; running up stairs; swimming with your arms while pulling a float board with your legs; or doing isometric contractions against an immovable object. But all of these share the common characteristic of adding resistance to the movements generated by skeletal muscles.

This book focuses on the use of free weights (barbell, dumbbells, and related equipment) and commonly available machines that are patterned after free-weight exercises. Whether you use free weights or machines to apply resistance, you will build strength.

STRENGTH TRAINING INCREASES SPEED

A large portion of speed in movement—sprinting, swinging a bat, swimming, skating, twisting, or any other sport—is genetically determined by things like bone length and the relative ratio between slow-twitch and fast-twitch muscle fibers (more on this in the next chapter). But speed *can* be improved through strength training.

The athlete's speed is related to his or her muscular strength. One reason is that a stronger muscle can more easily overcome resistance to movements, whether the resistance is gravity, water, or the added weight of equipment or implements.

Stronger legs are able to resist gravity more easily, resulting in longer, more frequent strides. In the same way, greater strength increases the speed of a racket, bat, or other implement.

Strength training won't turn you into an eight-flat 100-meter sprinter. (The record for men is 9.86 seconds, for women, 10.49 seconds.) The effect of strength training is limited by the parameters of your individual genetic ability. But you will improve your speed through strength training, getting the most from your body as you move closer to your personal genetic potential. And that improvement can mean the difference between first and second place, or between being tackled at the line of scrimmage and breaking away for the touchdown that wins the game and earns a league title for your team.

STRENGTH TRAINING INCREASES POWER

"Power back," "power hitter," and "power forward" are terms that conjure images of "powerful" athletes. But what is power?

As it arises in athletic performance, power is best described in terms of strength and speed. Whether punching, throwing, jumping, or batting, power is calculated by multiplying a movement's strength (force) by its speed: Power = Strength × Speed. Hence, through the powers of multiplication, an athlete's power increases when either his strength or speed increases. Since strength training increases both strength and speed, the result is a rapid increase of power.

The so-called power sports—football and track and field's throwing events—were the first to utilize strength training programs. That's because the association between increased strength and power is most noticeable in explosive movements such as shot-putting or the thrust of a lineman. But increased power benefits an array of explosive athletic movements from jumping for a rebound to batting a ball to the power of each sprint stride or swim stroke. And nothing builds power as rapidly as strength training.

STRENGTH TRAINING INCREASES FLEXIBILITY

To this day, it's not uncommon to encounter athletes or coaches fearful that weight training will create muscle-bound, inflexible athletes. This timeworn myth persists in spite of voluminous scientific studies and practical examples documenting that weight training actually *improves* flexibility.

The champion competitive bodybuilders at Gold's Gym are practical examples of the relationship between weights and flexibility. Top bodybuilders can easily touch their fingers to any point on their backs, and the majority of them can touch their palms flat on the floor with their legs straight, a feat few "average" individuals can accomplish. If champion bodybuilders can attain and maintain such flexibility through weight training, so can any athlete. Practical evidence comes from outside of Gold's too. A comparative study concluded that the flexibility of Olympic weight lifters was second only to gymnasts'.

As you can see, strength trained athletes are among the most flexible of human beings.

STRENGTH TRAINING PREVENTS AND/OR REDUCES SPORT INJURIES

Football players probably incur more injuries than any other group of athletes, but numerous college and professional football teams have documented dramatic *decreases* in injury rates among those athletes who engaged in serious preseason strength workouts.

The part weight training plays in reducing injuries can be demonstrated through the example of a weekend skiing enthusiast. Ski patrol statistics show that most accidents occur late in the day on what was intended to be the last run. With each run the skier becomes more fatigued, and with increased fatigue, less functional strength is available. On the last run, he or she hits a little mogul that might have had no effect earlier in the day, but this time the skier is too tired to handle the disruption, loses control, and tears up an ankle or a knee. If this same skier had had an excess of strength, the mogul would not have been such a threat. This same principle generalizes to all other sports. Extra strength is an insurance policy against injuries.

In addition to preventing injuries among serious athletes, a couple of strength workouts each week help prevent that oh-so-common Monday morning sore muscle syndrome that is the anathema of weekend athletes. And if you are a serious weekend athlete, these workouts will also give you a significant edge over most weekenders. You'll run a little faster, jump a little higher, win a little more often, and be none the worse for wear.

STRENGTH TRAINING MAINTAINS PRESEASON STRENGTH LEVELS DURING THE COMPETITIVE SEASON

As far back as the 1970s, a National Football League study revealed that athletes who did no strength training during the season lost substantial strength when compared to training-camp (preseason) strength levels. Players who managed one or two short workouts each week during the competitive season, however, maintained most of their preseason strength levels, and consequently had a higher level of performance than the group that did not weight train. That early NFL study has been verified numerous times since: all college and pro teams now conduct in-season strength training programs.

While it is practically impossible during the competitive season to participate in weight training sessions that are as long and intense as off-season sessions, an abbreviated in-season workout will *maintain* most of your preseason strength.

Maintaining strength demands less effort than adding strength. While it takes long, hard weight workouts to build strength, the experience at Gold's Gym has been that strength can be maintained with less-rigorous workouts. Two workouts a week consisting of 1 to 3 sets per muscle group, using 90 percent of preseason poundages, will maintain 95 percent of your functional strength over the course of the competitive season.

More about in-season workouts can be found in chapter 5 under "Seasonal Alterations" (page 66).

STRENGTH TRAINING CAN COEXIST WITH AN INCREASE, DECREASE, OR MAINTENANCE OF BODY WEIGHT

A strength training program, in conjunction with an appropriate diet, can be tailored to increase muscular body weight or increase strength levels without a body weight gain. Strength training programs can also be designed to maintain body weight over the course of a competitive season, something that is difficult for many athletes. Each of these goals can be reached with the strength training methods discussed in chapter 8 under "Selective Size Gains." Using these methods, a football player or shot-putter can gain the weight and strength necessary to reach excellence in their performance, and a gymnast or runner can increase strength without adding body weight.

SELECTIVE STRENGTH TRAINING CAN REINFORCE A WEAK LINK

An experienced athlete may reach a sticking point in his or her athletic performance because a single muscle group—or even a segment of a muscle—is too weak to synchronously perform with the rest of the body. Like a chain, your athletic performance is limited by its weakest link.

Strength training exercises can be chosen to stress a particular muscle group (or part of a muscle group) in virtual isolation from the rest of the body. For example, a rower with a weak lower back can choose exercises to strengthen the erector spinae muscles that cross the lower back, eliminating the weak point that blocks improved performance. Athletes can use selective exercise to rehabilitate an injured muscle. Briefly, a muscle left unstressed during the healing process will be significantly weaker than it was before being injured. Athletic performance suffers, returning to normal only when the injured muscle has been fully restored to preinjury strength. Consequently, selecting exercises specifically to strengthen the injured muscle will quicken the rehabilitation process, hastening the athlete's return to preinjury performance.

STRENGTH TRAINING WITH FREE WEIGHTS AND MACHINES ALLOWS A TOTAL RANGE OF RESISTANCE

If you have been using calisthenics—push-ups, knee bends, and the like—to improve your functional strength in a given muscle group, you know that the maximum resistance to any movement is limited by your body weight. But there is no limit to potential resistance when exercising with free weights or weight training machines.

Weight training equipment is weight adjustable, ranging from light to heavy resistance. You can load a barbell up to more than 1000 pounds—a weight that only an infinitesimally small percentage of athletes can exceed during any exercise. At the opposite end of the resistance continuum, machines and free weights permit a beginner to effectively exercise a muscle group with less than body weight.

THE MINIMAL DRAWBACKS OF STRENGTH TRAINING ARE EASILY MODIFIED

While there are many advantages to strength training, there are two potential drawbacks to consider. However, each can be avoided or minimized by following the recommendations in this book.

The first drawback is that strength training is repetitious, and you will be doing many of the same exercises thousands of times throughout your athletic career if you choose to weight train. This can lead to boredom and less-than-optimal workouts.

Boredom can be minimized by periodically changing the training routine. Frequently change the exercises, substituting exercises that work the same muscle groups. For example, switch from leg presses (page 98) to squats (page 92) to strengthen the muscles responsible for leg drive.

A second drawback is that, even though most athletes will merely redistribute their body weight while gaining strength, some will inevitably gain weight. Most athletes lose fat by expending extra calories during weight training at about the same rate they gain muscle. Thus, their body weight remains relatively constant. On the other hand, some athletes have a natural ability to gain muscle tissue. Many Gold's Gym bodybuilders would love to be in this position, but for an athlete it is important that weight gains be limited to functional muscle. For these athletes, the training procedures for selective size gains—gains in functional muscle—are explained in chapter 8.

• • •

Male or female, child or adult, weekend softball player or professional superstar, once you have made the decision to physically improve, strength training will enable you to reach that goal.

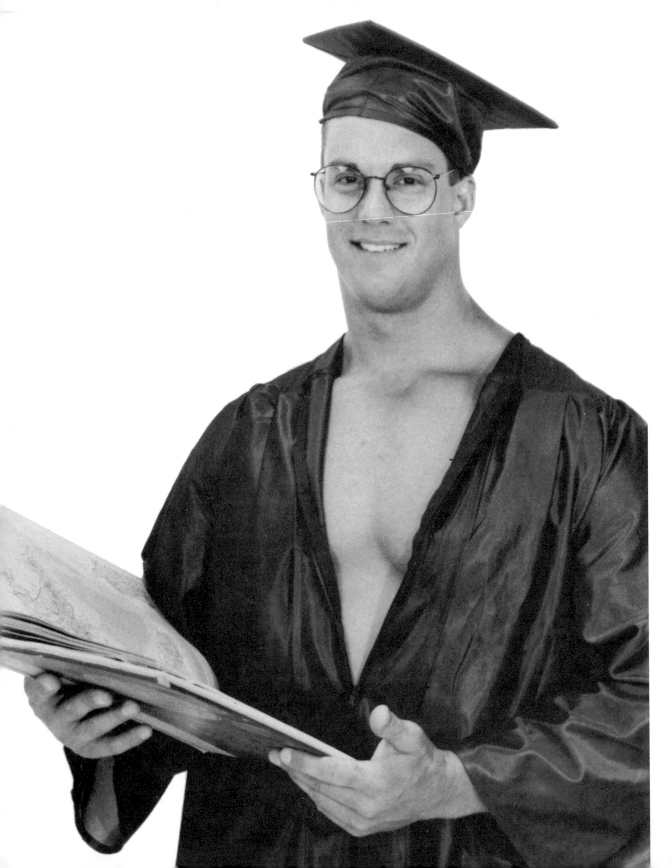

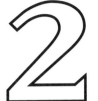

SCIENTIFIC BASIS OF STRENGTH TRAINING

> Science today is defined as the working out of naturalistic explanations for phenomena, and the most plausible naturalistic explanation is awarded the status of "scientific knowledge."
>
> Phillip C. Johnson, 1993
> *Los Angeles Times*

Science is a "best guess" woven from an interpretation of available evidence. That's the case whether the scientific discipline is rocket science or muscle physiology.

The word "science" comes from the Latin word *scire,* meaning to learn or to know. English custom defines the goal of science as an attempt to describe *how* and *why* things happen, without resorting to whimsy or magic for answers. You're interested in knowing how and why strength training results in strength gains and better athletic performance.

Since there is little research to rely upon, the science of strength training is based on a synthesis of discoveries from the fields of physiology and kinesiology. Until about 25 years ago, there was nothing systematic in training procedures, no two men trained exactly alike, and positive results were hit-and-miss. Men (weight rooms were male bastions at that time) who lifted heavier and heavier weights grew stronger as a result. But some men grew much stronger than others. That's about the time that serious researchers—physiologists and kinesiologists—began studying strength trained athletes to determine the best system for success.

Scientific Research?

There isn't a lot of scientific research that supports a link between strength training and becoming an elite athlete. How much is known? Consider the following:

1. The vast majority of people in strength training studies are average, sedentary, specifically disabled, or prisoners; subjects are rarely elite athletes.
2. Only in the past 10 years has any serious research been conducted concerning the effect of strength training on kids and adolescents. *No* research exists in which preadolescent athletes were subjected to the rigorous training schedules common among elite adult athletes.
3. Comparison studies of different resistance-training programs produce variable results, often due to the type of testing equipment used in the experiments.

PHYSIOLOGY AND KINESIOLOGY

Physiology is the biological science of all life processes, chemical activities, and functions. There are specialists in the field who study only work physiology or those body processes—such as muscle metabolism, oxygen utilization in muscles, and waste product removal—directly related to muscular work. Because strength training is directly related to muscular work, it is based on principles of exercise physiology, some of which you will learn about in this chapter.

The study of how the body functions under conditions of exercise stress began at the Harvard Fatigue Laboratory in 1926. The lab's first treadmill was driven by a streetcar motor that was only capable of running at four forward speeds and reverse. The lab dissolved in 1946, but in the 1960s the exercise physiologists who studied there later developed their own laboratories and departments of human performance on college campuses. Sports studies have expanded beyond physiology; motor learning, biomechanics, sports psychology, and sports sociology are subdisciplines of sports performance.

Kinesiology is the study of human movement, the mechanics of how muscles act upon joints. For example, the elbow bends because the biceps muscle contracts. The knee straightens because the quadriceps (front thigh muscle) contracts.

Kinesiological studies of muscle movement provide the rationale for the selection of exercises found in this book, but it is the physiologist—particularly the exercise physiologist—who has made the most recent contributions to strength training.

HOW MUSCLES BECOME STRONGER

The mechanism behind muscle contraction, a discovery made by exercise physiologists decades ago, is fundamental to understanding strength training. Without muscle contraction, there would be no body movement and consequently no need or ability to strength train.

Contraction means that the muscle shortens to produce the force necessary for movement. You can think of it as a rubber band working in reverse, shortening rather than stretching to produce tension. Each muscle cell in your body has this ability to shorten.

Many muscle cells contracting in unison produce the movement used for sports. For example, imagine contracting your biceps to bend your elbow. One end of your biceps muscle is attached to your upper arm bone, and the other end of the biceps is attached to a bone in your forearm. The elbow is merely a hinge in the middle of your bones. When your brain sends the signal, the cells of your biceps muscle contract: The contraction shortens the biceps, and your elbow bends.

Each of your body's muscles, such as the biceps, consists of hundreds of thousands of muscle cells that can—but don't always—contract in unison. Which leads us to what determines the strength of your biceps.

The strength of your biceps (or any other muscle) is determined by two factors:

1. The strength of the individual muscle cells
2. The number of the biceps cells that contract at any one time

When your biceps are working, the cells that contract exhibit an "all-or-nothing" phenomenon: that means that the cell either contracts with all possible force or doesn't contract at all. The number of your biceps' cells that contract depends on the work to be done—fewer of your biceps' cells contract when lifting a feather than when lifting a freezer.

That leads us to the next point: strength training builds strength in your biceps two ways. It strengthens individual muscle cells and it teaches more of your biceps' cells to take part in a contraction.

· Strengthening Your Individual Muscle Cells

Strengthening any of your individual muscle cells is accompanied by *observable* physical change. If you had "before and after" pictures of those stronger cells, you would find that:

1. The muscle cell increases in size. The larger size is the result of an increase in the number and size of the cell's contraction machinery (myofibrils);
2. More energy deposits, proteins, and enzymes are packed into the cell to support the additional contractile machinery.

Just as more pistons and fuel combine for a more powerful automobile, the bigger muscle cell and the extra biological fuel combine for a stronger, more powerful muscle cell.

You might want to know what many exercise physiologists theorize as the mechanism of muscle cell growth, since bigger muscle cells are inherently stronger muscle cells. (It gets deep, so hold on.)

In every muscle cell there is a dynamic balance between two kinds of body metabolism: *anabolism* (building up of tissue) and *catabolism* (breaking down of tissue). In short, that means that there is an ongoing tension between increasing or decreasing the size of muscle cells.

In most people, anabolism and catabolism are in equilibrium in a muscle cell. So, if someone has a daily anabolic rate of 25 units, he or she also has a catabolic rate of 25 units. Some people are slightly more anabolic or catabolic, and either build up muscle tissue or break it down. (Anabolic steroids gain their name from being growth-inducing hormones.)

By studying the muscle cell metabolites (waste products), physiologists have concluded that anabolism is apparently not increased when you are in an anabolic (muscle building) state as a result of strength training. Instead, your anabolic rate remains constant, but exercise will decrease your catabolic rate, yielding an apparent anabolic effect. In other words, rather than muscle building taking one step forward, then falling one step back, it continues to take one step forward, but falls back only half a step.

That complicated theory can be practically stated: strength training increases the size of a muscle cell by stimulating a change in the balance between anabolic and catabolic rates.

· Neural Adaptations: Training More of Your Muscle Cells to Contract

Just like attaching more tugboats to push or pull a river barge, recruiting more of your biceps' cells to contribute to a movement is another way to increase muscle strength.

Although they're perfectly capable of doing so, many of your biceps' cells don't take part in even your most intense efforts to bend your elbow. But they can be trained to contribute. The training increases communication with the nervous system.

The better communication between nerves and muscle cells is called *neural adaptation.*

Neural adaptations—not the increase in the size or strength of individual muscle cells—are responsible for the rapid strength increases during the first months of weight training.

What is the chain of events leading to neural adaptations? As noted above, the strength of a movement depends on the number and size of muscle cells called into action. The central nervous system (brain and spinal cord) computes strength requirements, whether threading a sewing needle or curling a dumbbell, and signals the correct number of muscle cells to complete the task.

Overloading the muscle when strength training sends a signal to the brain that more muscle cells are needed to comfortably complete the exercise movement. With repeated workouts, the brain sends the "contract" signal to the additional muscle cells. Like threading a needle, lifting heavier weights is perfected through practice.

Strength training stimulates the learning process, causing your brain to act like a giant switchboard, turning on millions of muscle cells that have always had the potential to strengthen a movement.

· Anabolic Steroids and Stronger Muscles

The size of a muscle contributes to the strength of a muscle, and anabolic steroids, coupled with strength training, accelerate the increase in the size of a muscle.

Under natural conditions (without synthetic steroids), there is an ongoing balance between the building-up (anabolic metabolism) and tearing-down (catabolic metabolism) of muscle. Through a complex hormonal response, strength training increases the size of an athlete's muscle by changing that balance, reducing the rate of muscle destruction (catabolic metabolism) while the rate of muscle buildup remains the same.

Testosterone Reduces the Potbelly

A new 9-month study by a Swedish research team found the following results with middle-aged men wearing a testosterone patch on their bellies:
1. Reduced waistline measurements of about an inch due to redistribution of the body's fat content
2. Reduced blood pressure and blood cholesterol

Although more research is needed to confirm the findings, the study makes intuitive sense because researchers have known for years that testosterone levels drop as the male gets older, causing more fat to accumulate. Increased levels of testosterone have the opposite effect.

Anabolic steroids have a different effect on the anabolic-catabolic balance. The steroids, a chemical compound equivalent to testosterone, increase the potential for anabolic (muscle-building) metabolism.

The increased anabolic rate combines with the reduced catabolic rate for rapid muscle growth; with the rapid muscle growth comes a rapid increase in strength.

GENDER AND AGE DIFFERENCES IN STRENGTH GAINS

As noted above, two factors can influence strength gains: an increase in the size and strength of individual muscle cells or neural factors that train more muscle cells to contribute to a movement. What does the gender and age of the athlete have to do with this?

Gender and age determine the amount of testosterone circulating through the body. And the amount of testosterone circulating through the body has a direct effect on the growth of muscle cells.

Testosterone is important to muscle growth because it turns on genetic switches within the cell's nucleus, activating the production of protein. Protein is the primary building block for new muscle tissue, so the body with more testosterone has the capacity to build more muscle.

Growth Hormone Builds Muscle Too

Human growth hormone (HGH) is a natural product produced by each of our bodies. As the name implies, HGH stimulates growth.

Throughout the past decade, many adult bodybuilders have been injecting HGH to enhance muscle growth. Interestingly, many physicians have prescribed HGH to healthy children [having normal amounts of HGH] during that period too.

Why? More than 10,000 children have been prescribed HGH by physicians to increase height. What effect it has on their present and future muscular development in association with strength training is anybody's guess.

Everybody—children and females included—has some amount of testosterone circulating through the bloodstream, but an adult male has the most circulating testosterone. That's why he has an advantage in building muscle and gaining strength.

The onset of adolescence in a boy between 12 and 15 brings with it a surge in testosterone production at least a thousand percent greater than during childhood, and at least a thousand percent greater than the amount of testosterone produced by the body of an average adult female.

Steroids, Women, and Children

Anabolic steroids, man-made chemical compounds similar to testosterone, build muscle. In combination with strength training, they increase the rate of muscle growth in women and children as well as in men.

For women and children, swallowing or injecting steroids creates the equivalent of a male testosterone factory inside the body. The body masculinizes, manifesting such things as a deeper voice and facial hair atypical to the average female or child.

What happens to the muscle cell? The muscle cell can't differentiate between the steroid and natural testosterone, so a steroid-treated muscle cell carries on metabolic activities and responds to strength training, much the same as a man's would.

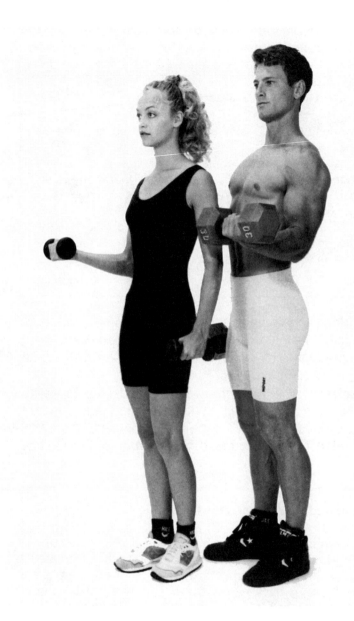

Because of their testosterone level, strength training produces a rate of muscle growth and increased strength attributable to muscle growth in men far greater than is possible for an equally trained woman or child.

Strength can also increase without muscle growth. The mechanism of these strength gains are the neural adaptations described above, and neural adaptations do not discriminate against age or gender. That's evident from the rapid strength gains made by females and children during the first few months of a strength training program.

Unfortunately, the rate of neural adaptations diminishes quickly, and further strength gains are closely tied to an increase in the size of the muscle. That's why the adult male athlete—with his high levels of muscle-building testosterone—has the greatest long-term effects from a strength training program.

STRENGTH AND TWO KINDS OF MUSCLE FIBERS

You're probably already aware that you have two types of muscle cells (also called muscle fibers), each with its own properties and each requiring a specific training approach for maximizing performance gains.

Your *fast-twitch fibers* have greater strength capacity, while *slow-twitch fibers* have greater endurance capacity. The focus of your strength training program should be fast-twitch fibers.

Fast-twitch fibers respond best to lower repetitions (in the range of 1 to 8) with a heavy weight, which is what I recommend here.

Scientists theorize that your genetically determined ratio between fast-twitch and slow-twitch fibers (everyone differs in fast-to-slow fiber ratio) determines your strength and speed potential. The greater your fast-twitch count, the greater your potential in sprinting and Olympic lifting. A preponderance of slow-twitch fibers increases your potential for running marathons.

· Determining Your Ratio of Fast- to Slow-Twitch Fibers

By this time a few of you should be at least a little curious to learn your twitch ratio. A muscle biopsy that counts the different fibers under a microscope is the most accurate method, but self-observation can provide you with a rough-estimate picture of your predominant fiber type.

If you have very little endurance and tremendous speed, your ratio leans toward fast-twitch, while little speed and excellent endurance will put you at the slow-twitch end. A few people have equal amounts of speed and endurance, about 50/50 fast/slow.

Strength training, especially if you are able to work out in a group, will also give you a good idea of where you stand. The sprinter types will progress very quickly in strength, while the marathoners will move forward more slowly.

Is strength training useless if you're a slow-twitch type? Not at all. Regardless of your twitch ratio, you can dramatically improve your overall strength through heavy-resistance training. And doing so will result in a more competitive athletic performance, whether you're a sprinter or marathoner.

STRENGTH-ENDURANCE CONTINUUM: A MATTER OF REPETITIONS

Exercise physiologists categorize athletic events according to the sorts of physical demands that the event places on the body. Strength, muscular endurance, and aerobic events are commonly used categories.

Events can be categorized by the number of sequential repetitions of muscular movements required to successfully complete the event.

A marathoner executes 20,000 sequential strides during the two-plus hours of the race. The shot-putter requires only one putting-movement during the fraction of a second that he or she powers across the circle. As you might suspect, the fewer the sequential repetitions required during competition, the greater the potential for strength training to improve athletic performance.

Success in movements like shot-putting, the thrust of an offensive lineman, or a tennis serve depends heavily on a single maximum muscular effort performed within a split second. Strength training has the greatest positive impact on these single-rep, maximum effort movements. Yes, the shot-putter, lineman, and tennis player make many duplicates of the same movement throughout competition, but there is a brief period of rest between the movements—time to allow muscles to recharge their strength potential.

The 200-meter sprint typifies what exercise physiologists describe as a muscular endurance event. That means it's dependent on numerous repetitions of near-maximum muscular contractions performed over periods of several seconds in two minutes. Strength training has a significant impact on performance in these events, too, because an increase in the strength of a muscle increases the number of repetitions the muscle can perform against a fixed resistance. A stronger leg can negotiate a hill more easily than a weaker leg because lifting the fixed weight of the body is easier.

The muscular endurance of specific muscles can be increased with high-rep sets (100 +) of any strength training exercise. But practical experience and research suggest that the athlete's gym-time is better spent training for absolute strength, allowing the increase in absolute strength to indirectly benefit muscular endurance during competition.

The marathon and other events demanding thousands of identical, uninterrupted, far-less-than-maximum movements benefit least of all from traditional strength-training programs. That doesn't mean that strength training should be totally ignored by the endurance athlete: the right program can prevent injuries or correct a weak link that might otherwise interfere with correct form.

In the age of cross-training, a point to remember is that maximal aerobic endurance and maximal strength are mutually exclusive qualities requiring markedly different training programs. Increased aerobic endurance and increased strength are brought about through different physiological changes to muscle tissue.

You can't concurrently maximize endurance and strength. While some individuals in superior physical condition appear to have maximized strength and aerobic endurance, they could attain vastly higher levels of one or the other by focusing their training time.

The best advice is to train for pure strength when in the gym. Let muscular endurance and aerobic endurance develop through the repetitions of practice and competition.

YOU'RE THE EXPERT

Regardless of the advice you get in this book, you are the expert on your body. You're the one who can digest all the information you can find on strength training and use it to develop a program that works best for you.

Your body is different from all others on this planet. You have different hormone levels, different tendon attachments, different recuperative capabilities—in general, a different genetic makeup—than anyone you know or have read about. Pay attention to yourself when designing or modifying a strength training program.

By getting in touch with your body, you'll be able to adapt the information in this book to suit your needs. Monitor your energy levels, strength-gain rate, fatigue-buildup rates, flexibility, perception of exercise intensity and pain, mental attitude, mood, pulse rate, and the feel of your body moving under resistance. Try to relate each of these factors to how you are progressing in your sport and you will develop a natural aptitude for training that will help you to progress more rapidly.

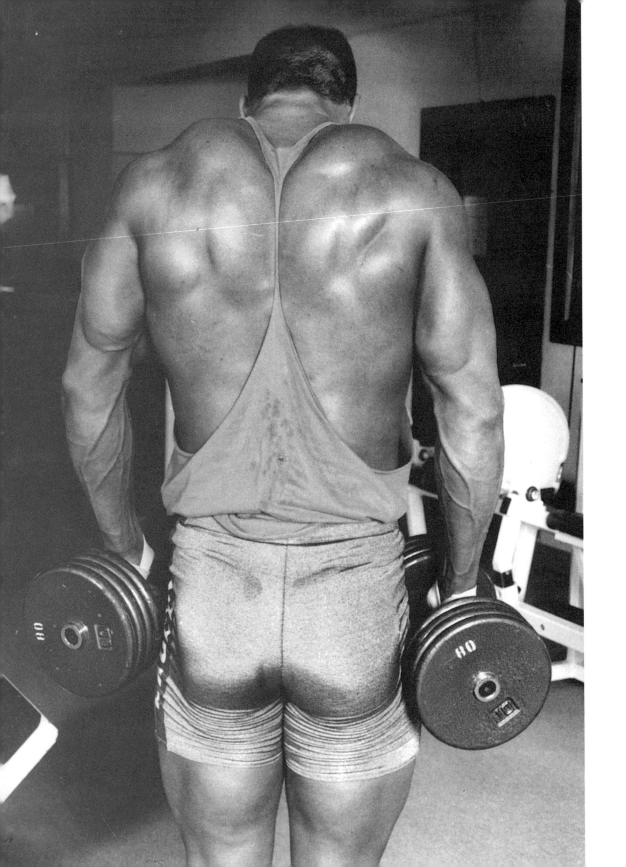

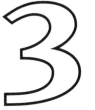

KEYS TO SUCCESS: SPECIFICITY, INTENSITY, AND REST

Strength training isn't rocket science. Add resistance to a natural movement such as raising your hand above your head or squatting toward the floor and, over time, the muscles controlling that movement adapt to the added resistance by growing stronger.

But there are three key factors at the foundation of every successful strength training program: they are intensity, rest, and specificity.

- *Intensity* is a measure of how hard you train. Training must be difficult (intense) enough to stimulate the muscle to grow stronger.
- *Rest* between training sessions must be adequate enough to allow the muscle time to recuperate from previous training demands.
- *Specificity* means selecting strength training exercises that closely copy your competition movements.

These three keys to success are all that stand between you and the markedly improved strength that will make you a faster, more powerful athlete.

As you read this chapter, keep the concepts of *specificity, intensity,* and *rest* at the front of your mind. Let's begin with specificity.

SPECIFICITY

Specificity refers to selecting strength training exercises that copy the movements of your sport.

A clear example of a strength training exercise utilizing the concept of specificity is a shot-putter working out with a heavier-than-competition-weight shot. Other examples are a softball pitcher rigging a weighted pulley to mimic a pitching motion; a swimmer pulling immobile legs through the water with arm strength alone; an archer practicing with a heavier-than-normal bow; a placekicker attaching extra weight to his foot; or a sprinter adding ankle weights. The common denominator here is that a sports movement is mimicked with greater-than-competition resistance.

Mimicking the movements of your sport during a strength training exercise requires a complicated two-step process:

1. The movements of your sport must be carefully analyzed and
2. Strength exercises must be created to mimic those movements.

As you might already suspect, many of the highly coordinated movements from the world of sports are virtually impossible to duplicate with standard strength training equipment. If you can't duplicate a sports movement in the weight room, what's the next-best alternative?

Selecting standard exercises that most closely duplicate the sports movement is the best alternative. That is the focus of the next section.

· Specificity Alternative: Selecting Standard Exercises

Specifically mimicking the movements of your sport is the best method of strength training. But when that's impossible, the best alternative is to select standard strength-training exercises that *most closely imitate* the most important movements of your sport.

Athletes have been using basic strength training movements for several decades. Football players build sports-functional strength with squats, an exercise motion that loosely imitates the lineman's drive off the line; boxers practice close-grip bench presses to loosely imitate a basic punching motion, strengthening the arm and shoulder muscles in the process; and dumbbell flies are substituted as a loosely disguised discus-throwing motion.

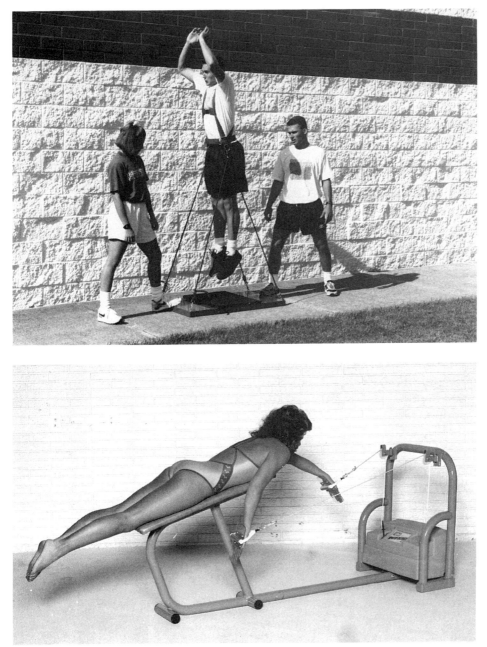

Specificity is sometimes best achieved with nontraditional equipment such as the pictured Velocity Jumper and Vasa Swim Trainer, which provide resistance to the athlete's natural competition motion.

None of the standard exercise movements noted above perfectly matches the competition motion. But much of the strength developed through the loose-copy standard exercise will transfer to the specific competition movement.

The typical strength-training program consists entirely of standard exercise movements. That's because program design is driven by available equipment, usually the traditional free weights and selectorized machines. Later, in chapter 8, you'll find tips on how to modify the standard exercises to more closely imitate the specific movements of your sport.

But for now, always remember that specificity is the ultimate goal in program design, exercise selection, and exercise execution.

INTENSITY

Intensity is a rough synonym for effort, how hard you train, how much you stress your muscles during an exercise or workout.

· Weight, Repetitions, and Intensity

If intensity is effort, how can we measure effort? You use the greatest effort (intensity) when performing the maximum possible number of repetitions with whatever weight is on the bar or machine. But there are limitations to the number of repetitions that optimize strength gains. You must select a weight that ensures that the number of repetitions achieved through all-out effort will not compromise optimal strength gains.

Although sets of anywhere from 1 to 12 repetitions have proven to promote strength gains, experience dictates that sets of 3 to 8 repetitions are the most physically and psychologically tolerable for the majority of athletes. Of course, the athlete will use a much heavier weight for a set of 3 reps than for a set of 8 reps. Regulating intensity is a balance between weight and reps.

As long as you operate within the parameters of 3 to 8 reps for each set—and that last rep is the absolute limit of your ability—you'll be using the correct balance between weight and reps to achieve maximum training intensity.

· Sets and Intensity

The number of sets performed during a workout is another measure of intensity. Five all-out sets rather than 1 all-out set of an exercise produce a greater training effect for a given muscle group.

The greater the number of sets, the greater the training intensity. But the majority of athletes have found through practical experience that 3 to 5 sets of each exercise works best. That practical experience corresponds to studies that show a leveling off of the rate of strength increase after the fifth set. That doesn't mean that 10 sets won't build greater strength than 3, but the rate of return for effort expended diminishes with each set past 5.

This means you should perform 3 to 5 sets of 6 reps for the greatest balance between strength gains and time spent in the gym. Remember to make each set a successful, maximum-intensity set by selecting a weight that ensures that the last rep, that sixth rep, of each set is the last possible rep.

· The Relationship Between Progressive Resistance and Intensity

Progressive resistance means lifting more weight during an exercise as you're able to do so.

As a traditional explanation of progressive resistance, let's consider your biceps as capable of curling 100 pounds on a regular basis. If we subjected the biceps to a load of 102 pounds, the load would feel heavy to you, but over time it would stimulate your biceps to adapt so that they would be able to handle 102 pounds regularly instead of the original 100. On the other hand, had you not increased the weight by 2 pounds, your biceps would remain at the ability level necessary to curl 100 pounds.

The reason biceps can either remain at the 100-pound level or adapt to the 102-pound level lies in the concept of equilibrium. An equilibrium exists between the strength of your muscles and the demands you regularly place on them. If the stress on muscles is constant, they will remain at a level of strength adequate to this stress. Most manual laborers do great amounts of physical work each day, but very few of them develop tremendous strength because their workload (sets, reps, and weight) remains relatively constant.

There is an equilibrium between work demands and muscle output. To overcome this equilibrium, it is necessary to progressively increase the demands in a strength workout. In our example, your biceps will adapt to accommodate 103 pounds of resistance if you stimulate a strength increase by placing 103 pounds of stress on them. And once your biceps are used to 103 pounds, you must immediately begin to use 104. By constantly increasing the resistance, you will stimulate your biceps to become progressively stronger.

Thus, it is only through progressively applied resistance increases that muscles continue to grow in strength. To achieve these increases in strength training through the concept of progressive resistance, you increase the reps, sets, or poundages for an exercise.

For example, if you're able to bench-press 100 pounds for 6 reps in a given workout, a week later you might be able to perform 7 reps with that same 100 pounds. In successive workouts, you have a choice: continue to use a hundred pounds until you are able to exceed your 8-rep intensity parameter, or increase the weight—say to 105 pounds—which will probably limit your rep count to 5 or 6. As you can see, the practical application of progressive resistance and maximum intensity are the same.

You are likely to be doing more than one set per exercise in your strength training program. As mentioned, practical considerations suggest 3 to 5 sets. So you will be trying to add one repetition or more to each set. And you should never add weight to the multiple sets until you reach the required number of reps on all the sets.

The ranges of reps you'll be given for programs in later chapters (for example, 80 pounds for 5 to 8 reps) are called *guide numbers*. In this example, 5 is the lower guide number—the minimum number of repetitions you should reach for each set. The upper guide number is 8, so you'll be seeking a weight that permits 5 to 8 reps each set. Keep in mind that as part of the progression, you'll be asked to do different rep ranges for different exercises, so stay alert to these guide numbers.

· Sore Muscles and Intensity

Whether digging postholes or strength training for the first time, there's no way to avoid sore muscles. Soreness is a natural result of more-intense-than-usual exercise.

Your consolation is that your body is a marvelously adaptable machine. It very quickly becomes accustomed to new exercises and won't become sore again unless you make another dramatic increase in the workload you are placing on the exercised muscles.

Most athletes find that a break-in period of light exercise-weights and low sets helps minimize the soreness. Your break might be an abbreviated workout. Just do one set of each exercise movement the first workout or two. Then gradually add weight and sets until you are up to the full workout.

If you do get terribly sore, the only reliable relief is a long, hot bath. The hot water increases blood circulation to those sore muscles, soothing the pain in the process. Other possible, but unproven, remedies include massage and heavy doses of vitamin C.

Soreness isn't the sole domain of the novice. The experienced strength trainer can also find himself or herself sore after a workout. As with the beginner, the cause is usually attributable to more-intense-than-usual demands being placed on the muscles, perhaps from a new exercise variation or an inexplicable dose of adrenaline that produced a superintense effort.

REST

· Rest Between Workouts

Rest between workouts permits time to repair microscopic tissue damage and restore energy reserves resulting from the intensity of the previous workout. For the typical athlete, workouts for the same muscle groups should be spaced 48 to 72 hours apart. That translates to the traditional advice of one or two days off between training sessions for the same muscle groups.

The need for rest between workouts varies from athlete to athlete, depending on the intensity of the workout and the athlete's experience, maturity, and physical condition.

Prepubescent and early-adolescent athletes tend to achieve greatest strength gains with a training schedule that includes rest days between each workout, perhaps because the abbreviated schedule permits greater concentration during actual workout times.

Adults run the gamut of effective training schedules. Some require two days between workouts. Others—such as experienced Olympic lifters—are able to train daily without detrimental side effects.

· Rest Between the Sport and Weight Room

Your strength workout can be at any time during the day, but it is best to have it at least two or three hours before or after your sports activity. Heavy work causes slight blood congestion in the muscles because heavier-than-normal circulation is necessary to remove fatigue toxins in the muscle and replace them with new fuel stores. This congestion is the famous "pump" the bodybuilders talk about so reverently. It lasts only an hour or two, but it does have a temporary tightening effect on the muscles, which can lessen muscle control. If you play basketball immediately after weight training, for example, your shooting touch will be off a little. It's better to wait a couple of hours for the pump to subside.

· Rest Between Sets

Last but not least, it's important in strength training to have a rest interval between sets. If you don't rest enough, you won't have your strength back for the next set. If you rest too much, you begin to cool off, which increases the risk of injury. Experience has shown that a 60-to-90-second rest interval works best for most people.

· Overtraining: A Symptom of Too Little Rest

Your body's maintenance machinery and energy reserves are much like your checking account. If withdrawals exceed deposits, you're going to go broke. For your body, this going broke is "overtraining," and it is representative of a negative balance between training and rest. A rule of thumb: if your muscles don't fully recover before the next workout, you're overtraining.

You can enhance your body's maintenance and growth through proper sleep and rest, a good diet, and workouts within your capacity. Train too intensely, too often, or lose too much sleep, and before you know it, you've overtrained.

A drop in performance is an indication of overtraining. It's what track coaches used to describe as "staleness." You'll also likely feel tired both emotionally and physically, and if you keep a record of it, your pulse rate will probably rise. You might experience a mild case of insomnia or a loss of appetite.

Overtraining can lead to injury as small stresses, accumulated over time, reach a breaking point. A muscle or tendon might tear or a bone might fracture.

The only way to stop overtraining before it stops you is to reserve the training-rest deficit. Start by taking a few days off: don't train in the weight room or participate in your sport. Follow this break with shorter workouts, more sleep, a better diet, and maybe a total change of workout routine.

Once your energy balance is back to normal, you can take a few precautions that'll lower the chances of overtraining again. Be regular in your diet and sleep, and be sure to progress slowly in the total number of sets you do during each workout. Perhaps reduce the number of workouts per week. You can train as hard as you want, but keep the length of your workouts down.

The point to remember is that each athlete has a distinct physiological makeup and a distinct tolerance to training. Hence, each athlete must set a workout schedule consistent with his or her individual makeup.

· **Sleep**

It's been said that each 24 hours is divided into three equal segments. The first 8 hours are for sleep, the second 8 for work, and the third for recreation. This is not true for athletes.

If you're an athlete with a regular job or a school schedule, you're actually "working" more than 8 hours when you add in your training time, so it stands to reason that you'll need more sleep than the average person. Unfortunately, your heavy schedule often leaves too little time for adequate sleep.

As a general rule, athletes are recommended to sleep between 8 and 9 hours a day, although some need up to 12. Try sleeping 8 or more hours at night and taking a short nap in the late afternoon. If you can't nap, at least lie down and rest your body. It'll recharge your batteries for the rest of the day and will help prevent overtraining.

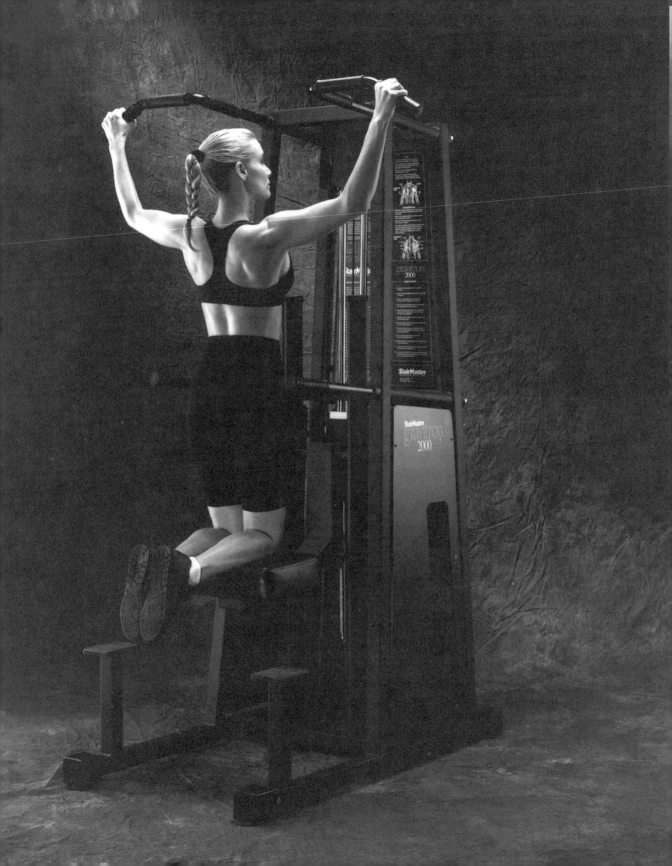

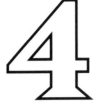

TIPS AND TECHNIQUES ON EQUIPMENT AND LOCATION

Your training environment—including equipment and location—has a direct impact on the success of your strength training program.

This chapter will acquaint you with facts and opinions about equipment and location to help you establish a positive strength-training environment.

EQUIPMENT

Above all else, choose the strength training equipment that allows you to most closely copy the athletic movements you want to strengthen.

All weight training machines and free weights will build strength, but maximizing your training time requires that you select the equipment that builds sport-specific strength. Reread chapter 3 if this concept is still puzzling.

There are practical limits to copying some of your athletic movements. If you had every piece of weight training equipment that was ever manufactured, you would still be unable to match many of your athletic movements. But your goal is always to match competition moves as closely as possible with the equipment at your disposal.

Let's begin our discussion of equipment selection with the oldest of the strength training tools: free weights.

Is Your Equipment Safe?

No single piece or manufacturer of equipment is best for all people. When making your equipment selections, there are considerations beyond price and quality of construction. Consider the following:

Size
Many pieces of equipment—benches, machines, and racks—don't fit all sizes of bodies. Body size, not age, is decisive. Fit can be unsafe for both the 4-foot child or the 7-foot superstar.

Experience
A machine exercise is usually easier to learn and easier to control than an equivalent free-weight exercise. Notwithstanding problems with fit, that makes the typical machine exercise safer for the beginner, whatever his or her age.

FREE WEIGHTS

Free weights include barbells, dumbbells, and related equipment, and are different from exercise machines such as Universal, Cybex, or Nautilus.

Barbells and dumbbells have been in existence for more than a century. Barbells are long bars with adjustable weights attached to each end. They're designed to be used with both hands. Dumbbells are shortened versions of a barbell (usually not more than a foot in length, as opposed to the 5- or 6-foot barbells), which are used as pairs, one in each hand.

A century ago, barbells and dumbbells were thick bars with solid iron spheres permanently attached to each end. Each barbell or dumbbell was limited to a single fixed poundage. Later the spheres were made hollow and openings provided in each so that lead shot could be added or removed, a crude method for adjusting the weight.

In 1902 Allan Calvert invented weighted disk barbells and dumbbells, the type still in general use. Almost a century of improvements have only altered his design slightly, and there is little difference between Calvert's adjustable barbell and the ones you will find in Gold's

Gym or your basement today. In addition, many commercial gyms like Gold's provide a full range of barbells and dumbbells with weights welded permanently in place. These "fixed weights," a conceptual throwback to the solid spheres, are a little more convenient than adjustable sets because no time is required to change plates on the end of the bar.

While barbell and dumbbell design has remained essentially the same, the expansion of ancillary equipment such as benches, pulleys, and racks enhances the application of strength-building resistance to all muscle groups. Through the combined use of all weight-related equipment, it is now possible to isolate resistance not only to a single muscle group but also to different parts of each group.

Benches have been built to place the body at various angles along a 180-degree arc from perfectly upright to head down in order to work with or against the downward pull of gravity. A variety of pulley arrangements has also been devised to circumvent gravity. The most common pulley device is known as a **lat machine**. It has a bar that can be pulled down from overhead to the neck, duplicating the movement and muscular activity of the common pull-up. This pulley-based lat machine, because it allows for a range of resistance from a mere 10 to hundreds of pounds, is useful for both athletes not strong enough or too strong to benefit from the regular pull-up.

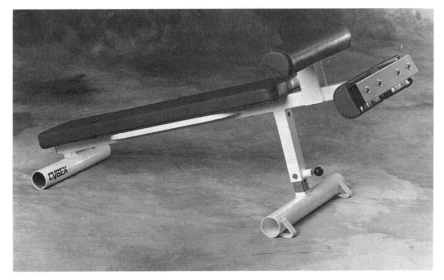

Adjustable decline bench

Squat rack

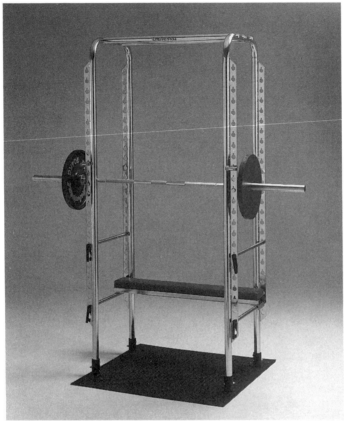

A **squat rack** is another common strength training device. There are many kinds of squat racks, but they all perform the same function—cradling a heavy weight at shoulder height. The rack allows you to perform a squat with a much heavier weight than you could normally bring to the starting position behind your neck. Can you imagine how hard it would be to get 300 or 400 pounds behind your neck without one?

FREE WEIGHTS OFFER THREE MAJOR ADVANTAGES OVER MACHINES

• First, they really are free, as in freedom. That is, they don't restrict natural body movements. You choose the range of movement with a free weight, and the barbell or dumbbell is merely along for the ride.

Conversely, a machine is a template for movement, dictating what you can or cannot do.

You control the movements of your body in your sport, so *you* should control the movements during strength training. No machine can duplicate the nuances of body control that allow you to catch a ball, run, change directions, accelerate explosively, or leap through the air for a slam dunk.

Comparing barbells and dumbbells, dumbbells allow greater freedom of movement and are usually better than barbells at duplicating the upper-body movements. The mere fact that barbells require the simultaneous use of both hands is in itself a limitation to copying the movements that you're likely to encounter in your sport. For example, how many times do you simultaneously throw a ball with each hand during the normal course of sporting events?

• The second advantage of free weights is economic, particularly if you train at home rather than at a commercial gym. Equipping a home gym with free weights and related equipment will cost you between $500 and $1000. That compares to the $100,000 or more it would cost to equip a home gym with the selectorized machines found in a commercial gym.

• The third advantage of free weights is the potential for a variety of exercise movements that machines can't match. Machines are limited in function, limited in the number of exercises—often only one, two or three—that can be safely performed for each body part. On the other hand, there are hundreds of free-weight movements for every muscle group. This variety of free-weight exercises reduces the potential for boredom that comes with month after month of the same exercise routine.

DISADVANTAGES OF FREE WEIGHTS

There are two disadvantages to using conventional weight-training equipment.

• The primary benefit of free weights—freedom of movement—increases the difficulty for beginning athletes to control a barbell or dumbbell. The difficulty is greatest during the first few workouts, when technique is being learned. But you can take solace in the fact that better control will soon come with practice, a fact any athlete has probably already learned on the playing field.

• The second disadvantage bears keeping in mind: machines are sometimes safer. If training alone, you're not going to be pinned under a chest-press machine, as could be the case when trying a 500-pound bench press with a barbell. Of course, trained spotters ensure that you won't have this problem with barbells. If you get stuck, they can lift a barbell off you.

Machines markedly reduce the number-one risk of injury in the weight room—dropping weights. But injury from a dropped weight most often results from two easily correctable causes: inexperience or trying a maximum lift without a spotter.

WEIGHT TRAINING MACHINES

With the growth of strength training has come the growth of strength training equipment. Barbells, dumbbells, and benches are no longer the only strength training devices available for home or commercial use. Hundreds of manufacturers have flooded the marketplace with machines to meet the public's heightened interest in weight training.

There are advantages to exercising with machines, safety being at the top of the list. But a strong functional disadvantage, as I have pointed out, is that machines control the body's movements. That makes mimicking a sports movement, the heart of building sport-specific strength, difficult to impossible.

Another functional disadvantage of multistation machines lies in the lack of variety of exercise options. Each station of a typical multistation machine allows few exercise choices. Given that strength training is repetitious, limiting the number of exercise options increases the probability of boredom. And boredom is the last thing an athlete needs for a successful workout!

We've already touched on economics of a machine-filled home gym: machines can be very expensive. Even an array of used machines costs many thousands of dollars more than new free weights and related equipment.

With that admittedly dour review, the following material is provided as a guide to the applicability of machines to your particular training situation.

· **Multistation Machines**

Multistation machines—ones with stations designed for different exercise movements—have really caught on the past few years in the home market. But they were originally designed for institutional use.

The earliest multistation machines, like the Universal Gym®, were marketed to commercial and school gyms. We had one at Gold's Gym as early as 1973, and it was in constant use. The primary advantage of a Universal-type machine is versatility in group situations. As many as 10 athletes can be on a single machine at one time, each at a different exercise station. An individual athlete's resistance level can be quickly accommodated with movable pins in each weight stack.

Multistation machines share the primary disadvantages of all machines: the machine controls the exercise movement, allowing neither individual biomechanical variation nor mimicking of a specific sports movement.

Universal® machine

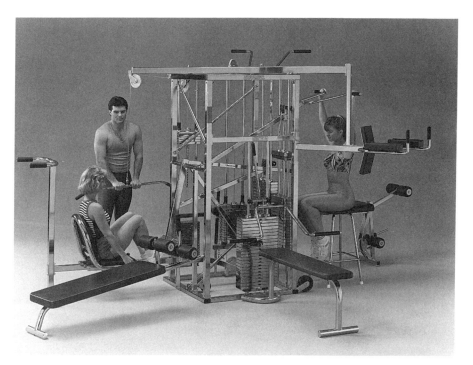

Soloflex® Home Unit

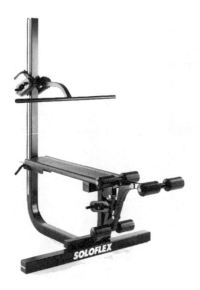

Is there a place for a multistation machine in your workout scheme? There certainly can be. A multistation machine contributes to strength development for all of the body's major muscle groups. The exercises may lack movement specificity, but so do most free-weight exercises.

Home units designed for numerous exercise movements have found a niche in the marketplace. An excellent example is the Soloflex® because of its capacity for adding barbell plates after the athlete's strength exceeds the maximum resistance supplied by the bands accompanying the machine.

· Single-Station Machines

Single-station machines—such as calf machines, chest-press machines, and leg-press machines—are designed to exercise a particular muscle group or movement. The popularity of single-station machines is greatest with athletic teams and commercial gymnasiums. Single-station machines have been a mainstay at Gold's Gym since the early 1970s.

Nautilus was the first big name in single-station machines, but other manufacturers have come and gone. The most popular among the current brands are Cybex®, Nautilus®, and Universal®. My son and I train with Cybex®.

Most single-station machines are designed to vary the resistance consistent with human strength curves: for example, the muscle's ability to apply force depends on joint angle. This is done by the cam-shaped pulleys that you'll often find placed between the applied muscular force (your hand on the bar) and the resistance (plate stack). The concept is grossly similar to balancing on a teeter-totter: force is determined by the distance the rider sits from the center. In the case of the machine, force is determined by the distance of the chain or cable from the center of the cam.

A machine that varies resistance at different joint angles offers a strength-building advantage. That's because the strength of a muscle overloaded throughout its full movement range will increase significantly more than a muscle overloaded through less than a full range. Varying the resistance throughout a movement is not possible with free weights: A 100-pound barbell is always a 100-pound barbell, regardless of joint angle.

Cybex® T-Bar row

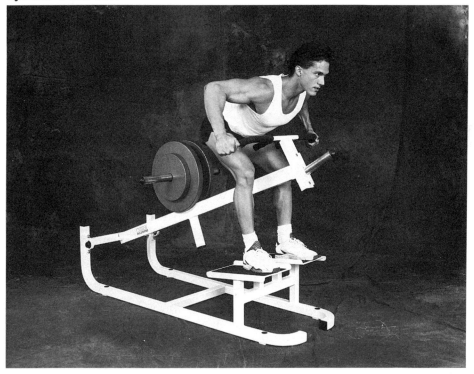

Once again, an obvious drawback of single-station machines for home use is expense. If you prefer single-station machines, best to join a commercial facility. Also, single-station machines limit potential exercise movements. For example, a leg-press machine permits leg presses and calf raises; scores of leg exercises can be performed with a set of free weights.

The final drawback to single-station machines is another familiar refrain: the lack of potential for specificity of movement so important to building sport-specific strength.

In conclusion, single-station machines, like multistation ones, build general strength in the muscle group being worked, provide a safety net for beginners, and are advantageous for team use since they run large numbers of athletes through a strength-training program in a short time. But machines rarely duplicate a sports-specific movement, and strengthening sports-specific movements has the greatest positive impact on the athlete's performance.

COMBINING FREE WEIGHTS AND MACHINES

Training in a facility where you can combine free weights and a wide selection of machines is the best of all strength training worlds.

A variety of exercise equipment offers a hedge against boredom as well as insurance that your muscles are being exercised through the widest array of movements. This is particularly important if you are unable to precisely duplicate a sports movement with one piece of equipment.

Working the same muscle group with a variety of equipment provides an umbrella, strengthening segments of a sport's specific movement too complicated to duplicate with one strength training exercise.

Accessibility to a wide range of equipment is tied to training location, our next topic.

WHERE TO WORK OUT

It would be insincere and a self-serving cliché if I were to write that it's not where you train, but how you train that matters. The truth is that training environment, including equipment, has a major impact on the success or failure of your strength training program.

Train where you have access to the greatest variety of equipment. That usually means a commercial gym. If you live in Los Angeles, join the original Gold's Gym—there's no better place. But don't despair if you're not an L.A. resident; there are other excellent strength-training facilities throughout the world.

When deciding where to train, consider a YMCA or school facility. Of course, these facilities vary widely in the quantity and quantity of equipment, and most leave you at the mercy of a clock. If you get off work at 10 P.M. and the Y closes at 9 P.M., you're out of luck. But if you find a school or Y weight room that's well equipped and open when you need it, such a facility can be ideal for hard athletic workouts.

If none of the aforementioned alternatives are available, or if you prefer privacy, open your own home gym. A positive aspect of home training is that the cost of setting up a garage or basement gym is a one-time expense, compared to yearly dues at a club or other facility. Another advantage is convenience, the chance to do some bench presses at 4 in the morning if you choose. The negatives of training exclusively in a home gym can be the lack of camaraderie of fellow gym members, a smaller selection of equipment with which to train, and faulty self-maintenance.

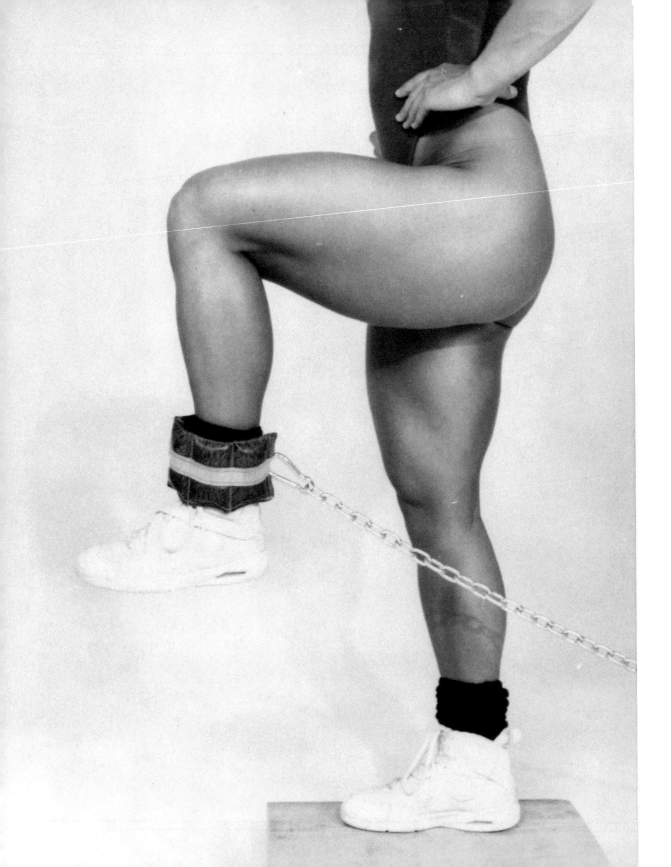

5

NONTRADITIONAL TRAINING TIPS

Weight rooms operate on tradition. Think back to when you walked into a weight room that very first time.

There was probably little rationale for your weight training program: you trained the way you trained because everyone in the gym trained more or less that way. Regardless of sport, size, or age, all of you trained as if you had identical strength needs. At least that's the way it was for me when I first started weight training more than 35 years ago in the basement of an inner-city YMCA.

Bodybuilding magazines are traditionbound too. The magazines' emphasis has always been—and continues to be—changes in appearance rather than function, still offering lots of advice on building big muscles, but little advice on how to put them to good use.

Although you may have been weight training for years, this book could be your first exposure to *weight training to improve athletic performance*. In this case the book is a "beginner's" book on strengthening movements.

Stronger movements make a better athlete. In building stronger movements, many of the traditional bodybuilding concepts that have been the foundation of your workouts will have to be cast aside.

NONTRADITIONAL APPROACH

Approach strength training with the four guidelines in mind:

1. Focus on building movement strength, not "showy" muscles.

2. Avoid traditional bodybuilding exercises such as concentration curls unless they strengthen movements important to your athletic event.

3. Ignore traditional bodybuilding concepts like high-rep sets of sit-ups that don't build strength.

4. Supersets, Tri-sets, Giant-sets—all bodybuilding protocols—have no place in strength-building programs.

Utilize your training energy and time for exercises and training concepts that add to your sports performance. In chapters 7 through 10, we'll discuss how you can determine which exercises are right for you and which to skip. Later in this chapter, we'll outline set and rep patterns that work best. But for now, read on with the above four guidelines in mind.

EXERCISE ORDER

Place the most important exercise at the beginning of the workout, and complete them before your energy and enthusiasm wane.

Reflecting the importance of leg drive and rotational force to your athletic success, train your legs and hips first, and trunk rotational muscles (abs, obliques) second. Train the chest, shoulders, and arms last.

· Train the Legs First

How big are your arms? How much can you bench-press? Whatever the psychodynamics, those are the most frequent queries in a weight room. But success in sports depends more on how much you can squat than how much you can bench-press.

A few facts: Throws and swings begin with leg drive. The force of each stride is dependent on leg strength, the height of each jump is dependent on leg strength, which brings home the point that the athlete must emphasize leg training.

Here are two practical tips to help you properly prioritize leg training:

1. Train the legs first during a workout. That includes specific leg exercises, such as squats, and ones that heavily involve the legs, such as power cleans and deadlifts.

2. Structure your workout so that 50 to 70 percent of your total

workout sets are exercises specifically for the legs or ones that heavily involve them.

Leg Exercises Build a Bigger Chest

If you need a stimulus greater than increased athletic performance to motivate your leg training, consider this: heavy leg work indirectly increases the size of the chest, shoulders, and arms.

How? Intense leg work, because so much muscle is being exercised, stimulates a temporary elevation of the blood level of growth hormone. And that increased concentration of growth hormone circulates through every capillary, interacting with the metabolic processes of each muscle cell.

That's one reason two athletes with identical upper-body training programs can exhibit markedly different results; the one following an intense leg program will show greater upper-body gains.

· Train Rotational Muscles Second

The abdominals and obliques, muscles responsible for trunk rotation, place a close second as "most neglected" in a typical strength training program.

Earlier in this book, you read that your muscles will grow stronger through progressive resistance training, i.e., training with ever-heavier weights as you're able to do so. Progressive resistance applies to all muscles, whether the quadriceps, pectorals, abdominals, or obliques.

Low reps with heavy weights builds strength. High-rep, low-weight sets do just the opposite, building endurance. But walk into any gym and you'll find most athletes engaging in high-rep, no-weight sets of abdominal exercises.

Is it important to have strong abs and obliques, the muscles responsible for trunk rotation? Michael Vessis, Ph.D., had this to say in the May 1993 issue of *Muscle and Fitness* magazine: "Up to 50 percent of the total force in throwing and hitting comes from trunk rotation."

Athletes also abandon the concept of specificity when exercising the abs and obliques. Yessis goes on to say that "Sit-ups do not develop these [rotational twisting] muscles effectively since a muscle should be strengthened in the same manner it will be utilized in an athletic event. Muscles such as the abdominals have more than one action, and if you develop only one action, other areas will be deficient." To develop rotational power, perform the reverse trunk twist (page 108) and twisting crunches and use the trunk rotator machines (page 110).

High-rep sets of sit-ups and leg raises are carryovers from bodybuilding magazines that mistakenly recommended hundreds of sit-ups as a means of spot reducing. Get modern and train your abs and obliques as you do your legs and chest—low reps, heavy weights, and specific movements.

REPTITIONS PER SET: 6

Heavy weights and low repetitions build strength. Light weights and high repetitions build muscular endurance.

Over the past quarter century, researchers have studied every number of repetitions per set in pursuit of an ideal rep-count. The practical solution: 6 repetitions per set, using a weight you can't lift a seventh time.

That's not to say that other rep counts don't build strength. In fact, research has demonstrated that anywhere from 1 to 10 reps per set will build strength. But for a multitude of practical factors, from safety to helping alleviate boredom, 6 reps per set is the ideal number for building strength.

There are exceptions: for example, after you've taken a few days off from training, then higher reps and lighter weights are best, but 6 reps per set is the cardinal rule of your ongoing strength program.

SETS PER EXERCISE: 3 TO 5

Studies have shown that anywhere from 1 to 10 sets of a given exercise build strength: the more sets, the greater the strength increase over the same period of time. That being the case, why don't I recommend 10 sets—or 20 sets?

Imagine the length of your workout and the potential for boredom and fatigue if you were to perform 10 sets of 10 different exercises during the same workout. A hundred sets. Your motivation would ebb before completing half a workout.

Why 3 to 5 sets? Because the return on investment peaks between 3 and 5. Yes, a sixth set builds more absolute strength than if you stop at 5, but the increment of strength gain will be less between the fifth and sixth set than the gain between the fourth and fifth sets. In other words, the rate of return diminishes with the increase in investment. It's like receiving less interest on the second hundred dollars of your bank account than you receive for the first hundred.

It's also okay to perform different numbers of sets of one exercise than another. The number of sets depends on the importance of the exercise to your athletic performance. Perhaps you'll choose 5 sets of squats and 3 sets of bench presses. The rule is that exercises providing the greatest benefit are allotted more sets.

EXERCISE POUNDAGES: HOW MUCH?

Resistance and reps are intractably intertwined. The general rule: select a weight that limits your rep count to 6. Err in weight selection on the *heavy* rather than the *light* side so that one less, rather than one more, rep is possible with the selected weight.

Is this safe advice? Yes, if you are following the safety precautions noted throughout this book regarding spotters, age appropriateness, and correct form.

· Selecting Starting Poundages

Everyone has a different strength level, so everyone will have different starting poundages. The following are broad suggestions on finding the starting poundage that's right for you.

To begin with, inexperienced male athletes should try one half of their body weight for all leg and back exercises and one fourth of their body weight for all other body parts when using a barbell or machine that uses both arms or legs. Halve the weight when the exercise, such as a dumbbell curl, employs only one appendage.

Lower levels of the male hormone testosterone will hold most women a little behind men in strength, so they should try two fifths of body weight for legs and back and one fifth for all the other body parts. Neither men nor women should use any weight at first for abdominal exercises.

From these you will need to decide if the weight is too heavy or too light and then adjust it accordingly for the next workout. Should you not complete the assigned number of repetitions, or complete them only with great difficulty, the weight is too heavy for you, and if you breeze through an exercise, the weight is too light.

Athletes with current weight-training experience generally have no difficulty deciding on an appropriate weight for a new exercise. For example, if they've used 80 pounds for barbell curls, they'll select 40 pounds in each hand (a total weight of 80 pounds) for dumbbell curls.

· Finding Your Maximum Weight

The topic of "maximum weights" comes up again and again in strength training.

A maximum single, also called one repetition maximum (1 RM), is the absolute heaviest weight with which you can perform one repetition of an exercise.

Determine your 1RM by warming up with lighter weights on a selected movement—for example, the bench press. After 2 or 3 sets of 8 to 10 repetitions with a light weight, jump up in 10-pound increments for singles at each weight until you finally fail and your spotter has to rescue you from being pinned under the weight. Your highest successful attempt is your maximum weight for that movement. Of course this poundage will go up as your strength increases, so most athletes will test their strength every 4 to 6 weeks. Testing more often than that can lead to overtraining.

Follow the same trial-and-error procedure when checking your maximum weight on a machine. What you'll probably find is that your 1RM on the machine is substantially different from the 1RM of an equivalent free-weight exercise. The point is that each should be treated as a separate exercise when deciding an appropriate 1RM.

Knowing your maximum weight has practical advantages in selecting poundages for your 6 repetition sets. That's because studies have demonstrated that the average person can perform 6 repetitions with 80 percent of his or her one-rep maximum. For example, if you can curl 100 pounds once, you can probably curl 80 pounds 6 times.

RAISING FREE WEIGHTS TO STARTING POSITIONS

In most instances, you will be able to simply pull or push barbells and dumbbells into the correct starting positions shown in the exercise photos and the descriptions that follow them.

The most important generalization to keep in mind is that your back remains straight and your hips remain lower than your shoulders when pulling any weight up from the floor. Initiate pulls from the floor with leg strength and then follow through with your back (i.e., straighten your legs first, and then your back when pulling).

With very hard weights, you can either take the barbell from the supporting rack, as for squats and bench presses, or have a training partner lift it into position for you. Either method works, but using a rack will be most helpful because sometimes you'll be training with partners who aren't available when you need them.

STRICT FORM

In regards to traditional exercises, swinging or "cheating" the weight through an exercise will lessen the resistance on some segment (joint angle) of an otherwise fully overloaded movement.

You will build stronger muscles capable of maximum performance through a full range of motion if you exercise your muscles through a full range of motion, taking care to extend the muscle to its maximum and then to flex it thoroughly. In other words, lengthen and shorten the muscle as much as possible.

Ensuring resistance over a full range of motion when using free weights or isotonic machines requires that you raise and lower the weight slowly and deliberately during each repetition—no bouncing or jerking. And lowering the weight under control makes the eccentric portion of your movement as valuable to your strength development as the concentric portion.

There will be times when "strict" form is not the same as traditional form. In other words, strict form in copying athletic movements might be quite different from the strict form as outlined in traditional exercise instructions. More on this topic can be found in chapter 8, under "Modify 'Strict' Form."

ALTERING TRAINING INTENSITY: WEEKLY AND SEASONALLY

Even one intense workout is both physically and emotionally demanding. That's why strength training programs are designed with safeguards to ensure that both the body and mind are ready, willing, and able to endure the months and years of continuous training.

· Weekly Alterations

The traditional training schedule developed over the past 50 years consists of 3 workouts per muscle group per week, each executed at a different level of intensity.

One weekly workout is high intensity (low reps, heavy weight, an all-out workout that stresses the body and mind to the max). One weekly workout is moderate intensity (medium reps, medium weight) and one low intensity (high reps, low weight).

The object of the traditionalists in varying the intensity of the workout is to allow for adequate rest and recovery. As you have read, adequate rest between workouts is a key to a successful strength-training program.

Given modern programs of 6-rep sets of maximum intensity, and the need for adequate rest, how should the athlete structure his or her workout week?

If 3 intense workouts per week won't allow adequate rest, consider lowering the frequency of workouts by training each body part no more than twice a week. Many champion athletes have excelled in strength gains with the twice-each-week, all-out schedule.

I recommend abandoning the traditional heavy-medium-light weekly schedule. Train as intensely as you can during each workout, as often as you can, as long as you respect the need for adequate rest.

· Seasonal Alterations: Periodization

Traditionally, athletes have followed instinct, taking time off or otherwise modifying training schedules when the intense stress of competition and training set off internal alarms.

My son, a shot-putter, added a practical spin when he said he needed a month off after "ten months of intense training for two days of competition" at the national championships.

Attempting to quantify instinct, exercise physiologists coined the term *periodization,* a pseudoscientific catch-all concept referring to seasonal changes in exercise selection, training volume, and training intensity.

Whether through instinct or science, periodic changes in the strength workout are necessary for three reasons: first, to avoid physically overtraining; second, to maintain enthusiasm, avoiding "training depression"; and third, to schedule yearly workouts so that the athlete's strength peaks at the peak of his or her competitive season.

The mind and body can't handle the relentless stress of maximum competition—or maximum training. Most athletes need periods of less activity between the demands of competition. That's one reason for the boxer's infrequent title defenses and for the off-season for basketball and football players.

Periodization is structured: a yearly periodization cycle is typically divided into 3 or 4 distinct training phases. If you function better on structure than instinct, I recommend dividing your yearly training cycle into the following 3 phases (seasons):

Preseason Training: The preseason is a time for strength and power building. The beginning of the preseason cycle is a good time to institute the Basic Movement Program outlined in chapter 7. As you adapt to the Basic Program, gradually add modifications suggested in chapter 8, Isolated Movements in chapter 9, or the Packaged Programs of chapter 10.

Since you'll probably be returning from a postseason layoff at the beginning of the preseason, the protocol for the first several weeks is sets of 8 to 12 reps, gradually returning to the intensity and resistance levels of the previous season.

Once back in shape, follow the recommended strength-building patterns of sets and reps outlined earlier in this chapter.

Competitive Season Training: The primary goal during the competition season is maintaining strength. The maintenance goal can be achieved with fewer sets (2) per workout, and fewer workouts (2) per week.

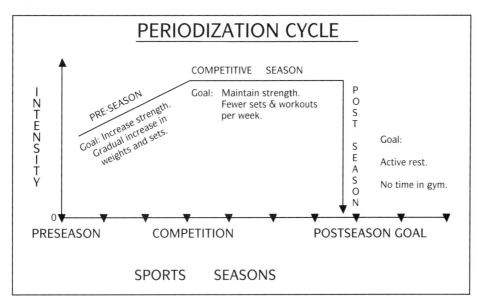

Postseason Training: The postseason is a time for "active rest": handball, cross-training, or pickup basketball games. Avoid any structured training, activity and play for at least a month.

Is a structured periodization schedule best for everyone? Probably not. Some athletes appear to work best without a schedule, relying instead on what Joe Weider coined as *instinctive training:* an intuitive synthesis of mind and body directing the intensity of training. As the competitive season nears, the athlete instinctively elevates training intensity. When he feels the need for time off, he takes time off.

The only drawback to instinctive training appears to be the greater likelihood of overtraining, of not being able to back off as the competition nears in order to marshal the physical and emotional artillery for the big throw or game. The instinctive trainer, out of fear of training too little, may lose his or her edge in the gym without the brakes supplied by a rigidly constructed schedule.

BREATHING

Trying to decide how to breathe during strength training can literally take your breath away. There are authorities who will tell you to breathe in as the weight is raised and out as it is lowered. Others say just the opposite. Numerous athletes have given each of these methods a fair trial, concluding that it makes little difference when you breathe.

Try each method and settle on the one that is most comfortable for you. Or, just breathe normally.

One caveat: don't hold your breath when performing heavy resistance exercises. Holding your breath involves what is called a Valsalva maneuver, a closure of the glottis against pressure, which interrupts venous return to the heart while raising thoracic blood pressure above safe levels.

MONITORING YOUR TRAINING PROGRAM

Strength training should be an interactive experience, responsive to personal feedback. You should cautiously experiment with new routines, equipment, and techniques to find an ideal personalized weight-training program.

When experimenting, consider giving your program a 6- to 8-week trial. This gives the program time to work. Keep written notes of the effects you achieve with different exercises and combinations of exercises.

When it's time to change routines, you can pick a new one from a later chapter in this book or devise a new routine using the advice in chapter 8.

A personalized program doesn't necessarily mean a complete overhaul. If you basically like your current program and are still making progress with it, try minor adaptations by substituting similar exercises for ones in your present routine. For example, you might substitute incline presses for bench presses, or squats for leg presses. Or it might be a simple change of grip or limb orientation.

· Training Diary

A practical way to look at your body's reactions is to keep a training diary. Enter the date, the exercises done, and the weight, sets, and reps for each movement. You may also want to include the time of day, your attitude, your pulse rates, the elapsed time for each workout, and so on. Any data you can include may prove helpful a few months or a few years down the road. From this data you can easily see exactly how you've reacted to the different exercises, routines, and techniques you've experimented with over a period of time.

The different routines and exercises can be cross-referenced with performance changes on the playing field to give you an integrated understanding of your total performance output.

Several recording codes exist for noting the weight, sets, and reps of an exercise. Below are several ways of saying 100 pounds for 5 sets of 6 reps of front squats:

$100/5 \times 6$
$100 \times 6 \times 6 \times 6 \times 6 \times 6$
$100/5/6$
$5 \times 6{:}100$

Any of these methods is acceptable if you can understand a year from now what you wrote down today. And don't forget to jot down your foot placement, hand placement, etc. Changes in body weight, aches and pains, missed days, anything. The more information that you record, the more chance you have of finding a pattern that contributes to success.

Good luck.

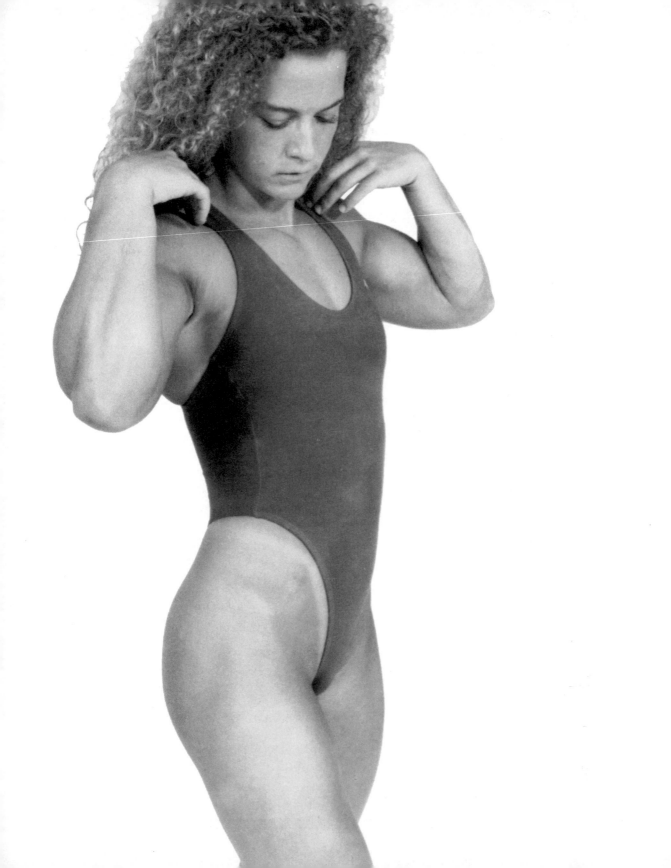

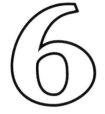

BASIC SAFETY, WARM-UPS, AND STRETCHES

Three or four times each year, my wife, son, and I climb into the family car and drive from our home in Oregon to visit relatives in Los Angeles.

Immediately upon arrival from one of those trips, my son, Chris—a 230-pound thirteen-year-old shot-putter with a competitive spirit—challenged his tournament-playing uncle to a tennis match.

"Ouch!" was the first word from Chris as he rolled over in his bed the next day. He had a terrible pain in his hip every time he moved. His back hurt, too. And when he finally stood, he limped toward the bathroom.

His injuries weren't serious—at least not to me—just soreness, a normal consequence of overdoing any new or unusual activity. And considering his competitive spirit, he was bound to overdo it.

Not every injury can be predicted or avoided, but the probability of serious injury can be reduced with a few simple precautions.

SAFETY FACTORS

There are important safety considerations covered elsewhere in the book. Check the following:
- Strength Training Reduces Injuries (page 19). Teams have documented decreases in injury rates among athletes who have engaged in preseason workouts.

- Sore Muscles (page 42). Sore muscles are a natural result of more-intense-than-usual exercise.
- Overtraining (page 44). Too much training and too little rest can lead to injury.
- Is Your Equipment Safe? (page 48). Not all equipment is safe for all bodies and all ages.
- Strict Form (pages 65 and 124). There are times when improper lifting technique can injure you.
- Rotator Cuff Exercises (page 174). A series of exercises that can help prevent serious shoulder injuries to an athlete whose event involves lots of throwing.

PHYSICAL EXAMINATIONS

You're probably tired of being told to have a physical exam before engaging in heavy physical activity. If you're like me, you wonder if the advice is at least in part an unnecessary transfer of wealth from your pocket to the gas tank of the doctor's new Mercedes.

On the other hand, there's the case of Jim Fixx, the author of *Running,* who strode his marvelously fit-looking body through a daily 6 miles. One day while on an easy jog, he keeled over from a heart attack brought on by clogged arteries that could have been detected with a routine physical. Jim is no longer with us.

At every level of scholastic sports participation, a physical examination is required, so many of you readers are already functioning within the guidelines. *If you participate in any sort of athletics without a physical, you are taking your life in your hands, especially if you are over 40*—Jim was in his early forties.

If you haven't had a physical recently, get one. Insist that a stress test EKG (electrocardiogram) be part of your exam. Some cardiac irregularities show up only under the intense stress produced in the treadmill test. Most authorities recommend such a test for persons over forty. We recommend one for serious athletes in *any* age group.

Swallow hard, pay the doctor. Yes, you might increase his or her standard of living, but you might also increase the length of yours.

COLLARS AND SPOTTERS

Sometimes we rebel against the simplest of safety precautions: many times in the past, laws to require seat belts have been resoundingly defeated at the ballot box.

That same sort of reluctance to follow safety precautions follows some of us into the weight room. It's a mistake because following two common safety procedures would eliminate the majority of all strength training injuries.

First check to see that the collars (the fastening devices on the outer ends of barbells and dumbbells that hold the plates in position) are in place and tightened. With limit weights, one end of a barbell will invariably go up faster than the other. If the collars are not in place or have not been tightened, the plates will slide off the lower end, and all hell breaks loose. A simple reach and snap will prevent that.

Second, have a spotter (or two) conscientiously attending when you use maximum poundages. Be especially sure to have one at the head of your bench when doing bench presses. You don't want your obituary to read, "a heavy barbell crashed across his throat while attempting his final bench press."

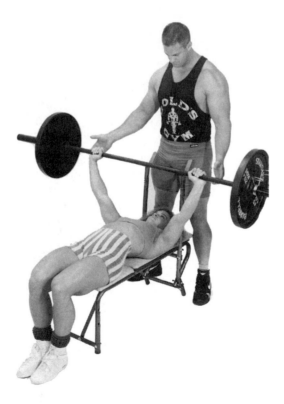

Spotter

· Training Partner–Spotter

The best way to be sure of a spotter is to train regularly with someone. Training partners can be motivational, too. You'll be less tempted to miss a workout, for example, if you know someone is waiting for you at the gym. And the natural rivalry that develops between partners leads to more dynamic workouts.

When choosing a partner, look for someone who is willing to follow the program you're on. Ideally, he or she should be in your sport at your approximate ability level. It will be more convenient if your partner is as strong as you are because you'll need to change weights less often. The final requirement is that the partner be dependable. You don't want to be left waiting at the gym.

Once you have a good training partner, use him or her to your advantage. By jumping in on exercises as fast as your partner finishes, you can speed up your workouts, which can indirectly build better cardiorespiratory fitness. And with your training partner as a regular spotter, you'll be able to force up your exercise poundages without fear of being stuck under heavier-than-normal weight.

SUPERVISING BEGINNERS AND KIDS

On the job or in the gym, the supervisor's primary mission is to provide guidance and direction as necessary to complete the task at hand. It's helpful having a knowledgeable supervisor prevent the pratfalls that can be anticipated only with the hindsight of experience.

Organizations such as the American Academy of Pediatrics and the National Strength and Conditioning Association recommend that kids (prepubescents) be closely monitored by an experienced supervisor when engaged in strength training activities.

The above caveat should be extended to beginners of any age. New activities—strength training to bicycling—carry unanticipated risks for the beginner. Safety precautions obvious to the experienced athlete are easily overlooked by the inexperienced athlete. In short, an experienced supervisor can provide a much-needed safety net.

This book offers great advice in print and pictures, but when a competent live supervisor is available, he or she can provide advice that can't be duplicated by any book.

Don't be embarrassed to interact with a competent instructor. You might be doing her a favor. If she's anything like me, her greatest insights into weight training will evolve from those interactions.

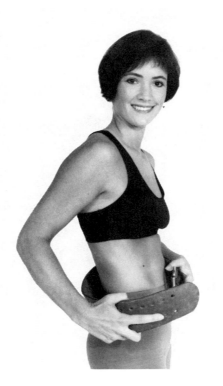

BELTS

Lifting belts—mechanical supports for the lower back and abdomen—originated with Olympic weight lifters. Many strength-trained athletes have followed the lifters' lead.

I'm undecided as to the overall value of a lifting belt. I never wore a belt during my competitive Olympic lifting days or when strength training for other athletic pursuits.

On the one hand, it does add support. On the other hand, by virtue of adding support—perhaps unnecessarily—it interferes with strength development of the very muscles it supports. Of course, it can't be worn during competition, when your back and abdomen are under the greatest stress.

If you choose to wear a belt, find one that's fitted to your waist measurement. If available, a 6-inch-wide belt is recommended for athletes over 5'8" and a 4-inch-wide belt for those under 5'8".

You should use the belt on all movements in which your back is not supported by weight apparatus—that includes all standing lifts.

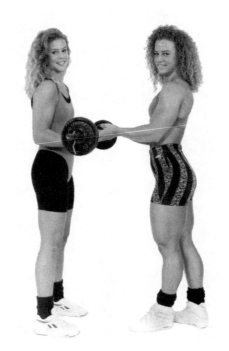

SAFE TRAINING LEVEL

Each person who picks up this book should begin strength training at the correct level. If you are a beginner, there's no problem, because you can open the book to the first page and progress straight through. If you have had some strength training, however, you will need some guidelines on where to begin again.

If you can remember the last time you did some strength work and can recall approximately how many total sets you did with each workout, it will be easy to give you a good general guideline for your re-entry level. If you've been off 6 months or less, do 50 percent of the total number of sets you used to do for your first workout, and use a poundage approximately 50 percent less than you used to handle in each movement. If you've been off more than 6 months, try a 33/33 formula instead of 50/50. Either way, work up slowly in both sets and poundages.

If you can't remember your sets and poundages and you've done 3 months or less of weight workouts, train as a beginner. If you've had 3 to 6 months of weight workouts, begin at Level One (chapter 7) or Packaged Sports Programs (chapter 10).

Pain, A Signal To Stop

Sharp pain is a signal to stop exercising: immediately! Whether running, throwing, or lifting, "no pain, no gain" does not apply to sudden sharp pain. Unlike minor soreness, a sharp, suddenly occurring pain can indicate a serious injury. Training through the pain can exacerbate an injury. Stop—and consult with a physician if the pain persists.

WARM UP FOR SAFETY AND PERFORMANCE

A survey of gym owners suggests that fewer than 10 percent of the members engage in a systematic full-body warm-up before weight training. Is a general warm-up a benefit?

The world of sports offers an easily digestible answer. Before Michael Jordan walks onto the court for a game, he warms up with a series of pregame drills to prepare his body for the all-out effort of competition. That's also the case for boxers, football players, baseball players, hurdlers, and so on. Universally, in the world of sports, a warm-up is a prelude to intense effort—benefiting the athlete by increasing capacity for strength and endurance while lowering the risk of injury.

In many ways, the all-out effort of strength training will be more intense than anything you've ever done. The muscles are working at maximum capacity. I strongly recommend that you follow the lead of your fellow athletes and warm up before doing any heavy-resistance work.

The warm-up produces at least two measurable physiological changes in the muscle and connective tissue. The warm-up raises the temperature of the muscles. The higher temperature contributes to an increased rate of chemical reactions and the greater strength and endurance capacity.

The increased activity of the warm-up exercises produces a corresponding increase in the amount of synovial fluid in the joint and an increase in the blood flow to the specific muscles involved in the exercise activity.

The best advice for warm-ups prior to strength training?

1. Ten minutes of your choice of a moderate aerobic activity. Perhaps punching a heavy bag, jogging in place, or using a rowing machine.

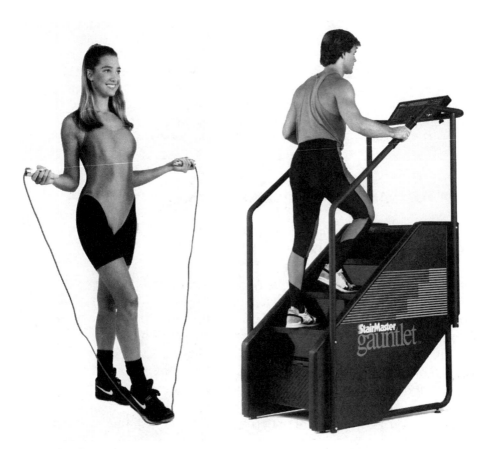

2. Supplemental movements—back bend, shoulder rolls, head rolls—for specific areas neglected during general warm-up activities.

3. One set of 15 repetitions of each strength training exercise performed immediately before the intense sets of that exercise.

STRETCH AFTER STRENGTH TRAINING

Warm-up exercises and stretches are different, and they should be performed at different points of the workout. The warm-up precedes strength training; stretching follows.

The focus of stretching is flexibility. The focus of the warm-up is to prepare for intense muscular stress. Don't confuse one with the other. And don't alter the sequence: if you stretch for your warm-up, your muscles are ill-prepared for intense effort, and your potential for injury rises. Best to raise the temperature of your muscles and reduce the potential for injury.

Stretches are valuable tools for the strength trainer. Studies indicate that stretching included as part of an overall workout program increases the strength of the affected muscles.

The safest and most effective time to stretch is following the workout, when your muscles are warm and pliable and the potential for injury is reduced.

Warm-up Routine

A "no-equipment" warm-up could be:

Cardiovascular Warm-up
Any combination of 10 minutes of the following:
· Jumping rope · Jogging or marching in place
· Stair climber · Heavy punching bag · Treadmill · Exercycle

Additional Movements
· Head rolls
· Shoulder rolls
· Twisting with a stick
· Floor touch/back roll-ups
· Calf stretch

Many books dealing with warm-ups are available. If you would prefer warm-up and stretching routines other than the ones detailed here, try Hyman Jampol's *The Weekend Athlete's Way to a Pain-Free Monday,* Bob Anderson's *Stretching,* and Michael Alter's *Sport Stretch.*

· **How to Stretch**

1. Gradually assume a stretch, easing toward the point of maximum tension, never extending the joint beyond a point of discomfort.

2. Never bounce. In addition to increasing the potential for injury, bouncing activates what is called the stretch reflex mechanism. This limits the range of any stretch, making it less effective.

3. Hold the stretch for 15 to 30 seconds, breathing steadily, and slowly release. Repeat if desired.

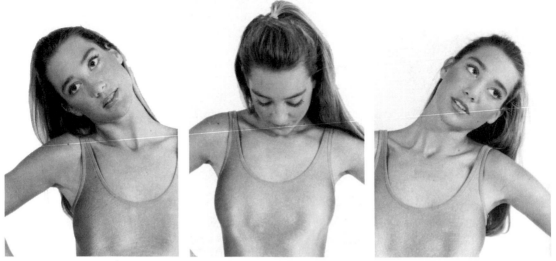

Head rolls Gently roll your head, tipping your left ear toward your left shoulder, then tipping your chin down toward your chest, and finally tipping your right ear toward your right shoulder. Reverse the direction and repeat three times without jerking your neck.

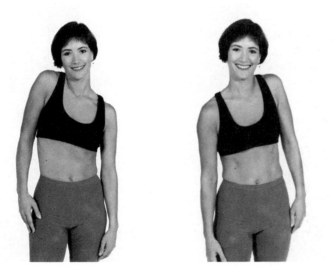

Shoulder rolls Stand with your feet apart. Alternate rolling each shoulder forward and back in small circles. Roll several times and feel your muscles across your upper back warm up.

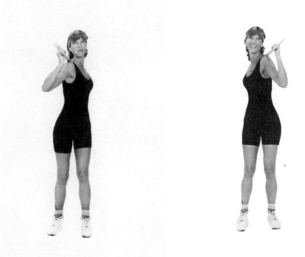

Twisting with stick Place an unloaded exercise bar or a stick across your shoulders in back of your neck. Facing straight forward, twist rhythmically and smoothly from side to side for several minutes.

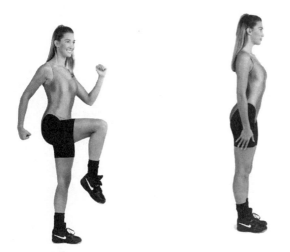

Marching in place March in place, emphasizing high knee action to warm your gluteals, hamstrings, and hip flexors.

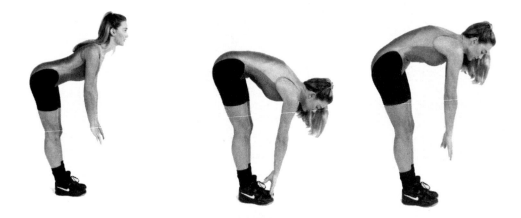

Back roll Stand with your feet shoulder-width apart. Reach toward your toes, maintaining an arched back as long as possible, rounding your back as you near the floor. Return by rolling upward to the starting position.

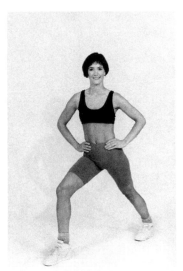

Calf stretch Place your right foot forward and your left foot back with your heel flat on the floor. Keep your left knee locked and your body weight forward. Alternate sides after 30 to 60 seconds.

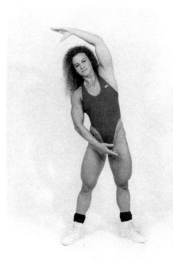

Overhead side stretch
Stretches the entire
side of the torso.

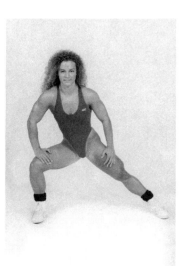

Side leg stretch Stretches
your inner thighs
and hamstrings.

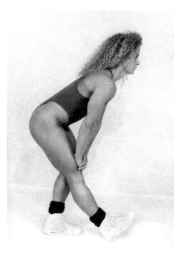

Front leg stretch
Stretches your calves,
Achilles, and hamstrings.

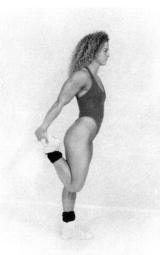

Quadriceps stretch
Stretches the quadriceps
and hip flexors.

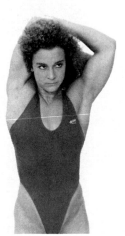
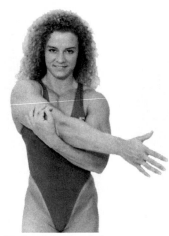

Triceps stretch Stretches the triceps and shoulder muscles.

Deltoid stretch Stretches the upper-back muscles as well as the deltoid.

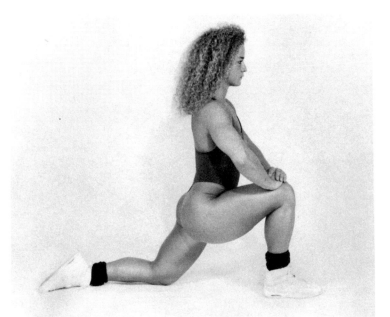

Kneeling stretch Stretches the gluteals, hip flexors, Achilles, and quadriceps.

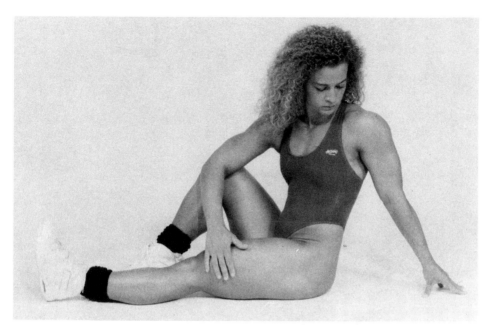

Seated trunk stretch Stretches the hips, obliques, lower-back muscles, gluteals, and neck muscles.

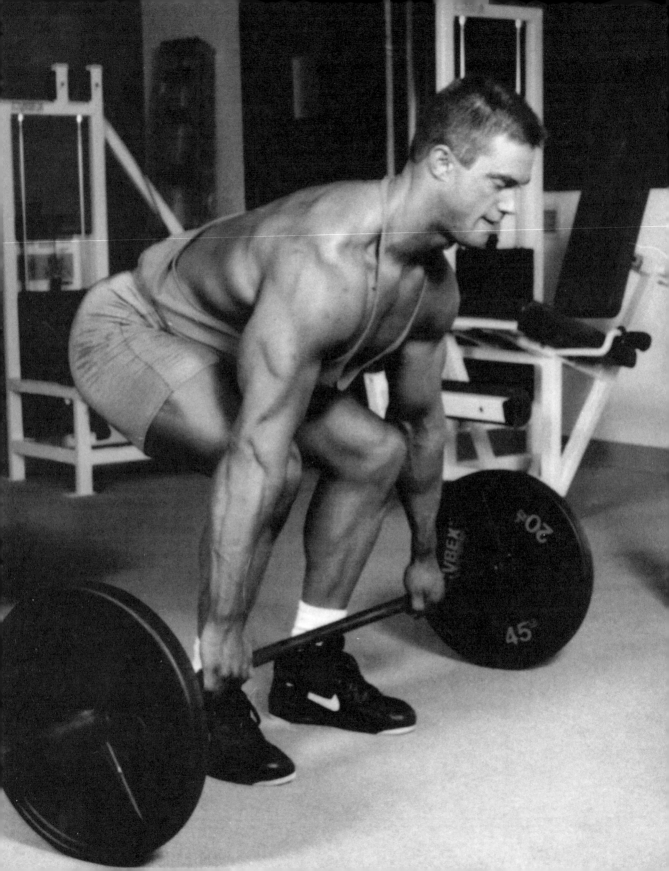

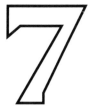

Level One: The Basic Movement Program

Your body's 206 bones and 400 skeletal muscles combine for millions of subtly different athletic movements, and strengthening those muscles and bones improves your capacity to move. But even if you're the most dedicated athlete in the weight room, you don't have the time or equipment to strengthen every specific motion your sport involves. What's the solution?

The solution is the Basic Movement Program, a manageable group of 5 exercises that strengthen the 5 basic athletic movements common to most sports.

The Basic Movement Program is not an "easy" program—some of the exercises are among the most demanding that you'll encounter throughout your strength training career. That's because each exercise works lots of muscles—demanding lots of effort and power output.

The 5 exercises of the Basic Movement Program work each of your body's major muscle groups: chest, back, shoulders, arms, abdominals, thighs, and calves. That's a bonus for a 5-exercise workout.

WHAT ARE THE 5 BASIC MOVEMENTS?

The 5 Basic Movements are:

- Leg Drive
- Pull
- Knee Lift
- Trunk Rotation
- Push

The countless twists, turns, leaps, and thrusts that are part of the athlete's event technique—decathelete, basketball player, or sumo wrestler—are based on these 5 basic movements.

To appreciate that point, consider the similarity of the leg drive of the high jumper, shot-putter, and sprinter. Each athlete uses the same muscles acting in a similar manner to extend the leg, driving the body forward or upward. Yes, each athlete has refined the leg drive to meet the technical demands of his particular sport. But regardless of technique, the movement retains the fundamental character of a "basic" leg drive, powered by the same muscles of the leg and hips and acting through the same joints on the same bones.

Trunk rotation is the same basic movement for the baseball batter, football passer, boxer, tennis player, or discus thrower. The muscles of the abdominals, obliques, and back twist the trunk, creating the rotational force that is ultimately transferred to the bat, ball, glove, racquet, or discus. The similarity extends to all movements, all athletes, and all sports.

The Basic Movement Program will be of considerable value in improving your sports performance, and you'll begin noticing results almost immediately.

Why Use the Basic Program?

The Beginner
The Basic Program is recommended as a 6-week stand-alone program for building a full–body strength foundation before moving on to chapters 8, 9, and 10.

The Advanced Strength Trainer
The Basic Program is recommended for anyone returning from a layoff; as the preseason cycle of a periodization schedule (see page 66); and the core of a sport-specific packaged program (see page 179).

The Team
The Basic Program offers a time-managed structured system convenient for the coach and athlete. The exercises are the same for the beginner or advanced athlete; only the sets, reps, and weights are changed to fit individual ability level.

WHY THESE EXERCISES?

The exercises for the Basic Movement Program were selected for one purpose: each exercise strengthens one of the 5 basic movements.

An added benefit is that all of the selected exercises use multiple muscle groups in concert to move the weight. For example, the bench press relies on the pectorals, deltoids, triceps, and, to a lesser degree, the latissimus dorsi and forearm muscles. The dumbbell press works the deltoids, triceps, and trapezius, while the squat works front thigh, hamstrings, calves, erector spinae, and trapezius.

HOW ARE THE BASIC PROGRAM EXERCISES GROUPED?

The exercises are grouped by the Basic Movement that is being strengthened. All the exercises that strengthen the Leg Drive are grouped together; all the exercises that strengthen the Push are grouped together; and so on.

For example, the squat strengthens the Leg Drive. It is grouped with the lunge, leg press, step-ups and other exercises that strengthen the Leg Drive.

Why is grouping important? With help from the Program Template below, grouping the exercises allows you to design your own Basic Movement Program, while ensuring selection of a complete, full-body, 5-movement workout. By group, the following are the Basic Program free weight and machine equivalent exercises:

	Free-Weight Exercise	**Machine Exercise**
Leg Drive		
	Squat	
	Front squat	Hack squat
	Lunge	Leg press
	Step-ups	
Pull		
	Power cleans	
	High pull	
	Deadlift	Seated cable long pull

	Free-Weight Exercise (cont.)	**Machine Exercise** (cont.)
Knee Lift		
	Leg raises	
	Hanging leg raises	
	Frog kicks	Knee lift w/pulley
Trunk Rotation		
	Reverse trunk twist	Rotary torso
Push		
	Barbell push press	
	Dumbbell push press	
	Alternating dumbbell push press	

BEFORE ATTEMPTING ANY EXERCISE

Before attempting any free-weight exercise, thoroughly read the instructions in this book, with particular attention to the Biomechanical Tips that follow each exercise. These tips contain safety precautions as well as indications of the physiological benefits of the exercise.

If you're training with a machine rather than free weights, read the manufacturer's instructions before trying to operate the machine. Instructions are often mounted on the machine for your convenience.

YOUR BASIC MOVEMENT PROGRAM

The Basic Movement Program is actually 576 different programs. That's how many different 5-movement exercise combinations are possible from the 19 different exercises.

But the elegance of the program requires that you select only 5 exercises: one for each of 5 Basic Movements. Combined, those 5 exercises will build a strength foundation for any athlete.

The Program Chart below makes it easy. You just choose one exercise from each of the Basic Movement groups.

THE PROGRAM CHART

The Program Chart is your training schedule. Simply select one exercise from each Basic Movement category and write that exercise into the appropriate spot on your Program Chart.

You're ready to train. Follow the exercise instructions for the exercises that you've selected, and follow the weight, set, and rep suggestions on the Program Chart.

The following are sample selections from the 5 Basic Movement categories. Charts that you can photocopy and fill in as you select your 5 Basic Movement exercises.

The Basic Program will improve any athlete's sports performance, and he or she will begin noticing results almost immediately. However, if you have had immediate prior strength-training experience and you are accomplished in the exercises in the Basic Program, you are probably ready to address the strength requirements specific to your sport. In that case, turn to chapter 10 for a Packaged Sports Program. Or you may want to develop your own program with the advice offered in chapters 8 and 9.

Otherwise it's time to select exercises, fit them into your Program Chart, and train.

NAME			WORKOUT		CHART	
	DATE	WEIGHT	SETS	REPS	Notes	Comments
LEG DRIVE						
PULL						
KNEE LIFT						
TRUNK ROTATION						
PUSH						
SPECIALTY EXERCISES*						

*Fill in after reading chapters 7 and 8.

BASIC MOVEMENT EXERCISE DESCRIPTIONS

BASIC MOVEMENT ONE: LEG DRIVE

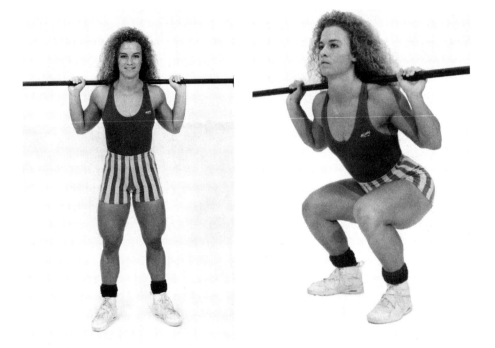

SQUAT

Muscles Involved
The front thighs and gluteal muscles of the buttocks, with secondary emphasis on the hamstrings, lower back, and the supporting muscles of the abdomen.

Barbell Starting Position
Stand erect with your feet about shoulder-width apart and your toes pointed slightly outward. Place a barbell across your shoulders and behind your neck, centering it and balancing it in place by grasping the bar with your hands out near the plates, palms facing forward. Keep your body upright throughout the movement.

Performance
1. Bend your knees and sink down in a deep knee-bend until your thighs are parallel to the floor.
2. Return to the upright position.
3. Repeat as required.

Note: With light weights you will be able to place the bar behind your neck with arm strength, but as you progress it will be best to load up the barbell on a squat rack and take it off the rack for each set.

Biomechanical Tips
Never bounce at the bottom of any squatting movement. This puts exceptional strain on your knee ligaments and your lower back. Never bend over at the waist during any part of the movement. This can injure your lower back. To keep your torso upright, pick a focus point for your eyes and keep looking at it as you squat down and come back up. This will keep your head up, which will in turn keep your torso upright. If you have difficulty keeping your feet flat on the floor, rest your heels on a 2 × 4-inch board.

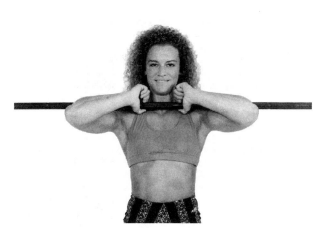

Variation: Front Squat Performance

Stand erect with your feet about shoulder-width apart and your toes pointed slightly outward. Hold a barbell in front of your neck and across your deltoids, steadying it with your hands toward the middle of the barbell, elbows at shoulder level. Tighten all of your back muscles.

Biomechanical Tips

Keep your torso perfectly upright to avoid straining your lower back. Also, if you bend forward while squatting, you will no doubt dump the bar off your shoulders and onto the floor.

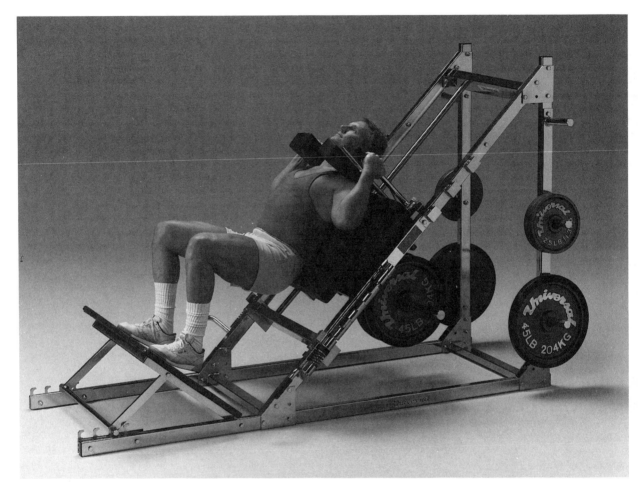

HACK SQUAT

Muscles Involved

The quadriceps at the fronts of the thighs, and the gluteals.

Biomechanical Tip

Correct foot placement on the footpad depends on leg length. Taller athletes position the feet toward the front of the footpad, shorter athletes toward the back. The object of foot placement is to minimize knee stress when your thigh is perpendicular to the footpad—the low position of the exercise.

Correct Technique

1. Facing away from the machine, position your shoulders under the shoulder pads, pressing your back against the back pad.

2. Stand erect while releasing safety stops at the side of the machine.

3. Breathe in as you lower your body until your thighs are parallel to the footpad.

4. With back pressed against the back pad, hold your breath as you return to the standing position. Release your breath at the top. That's a rep.

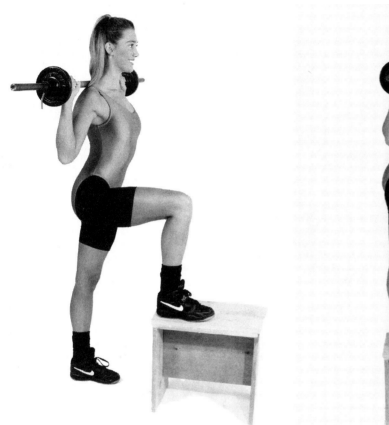
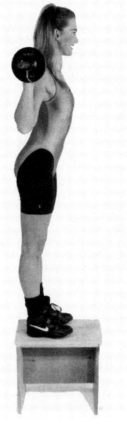

STEP-UPS

Muscles Involved
The quadriceps at the fronts of the thighs and the gluteal muscles of the buttocks, with secondary emphasis on the hip flexors, hamstrings, lower back, calves, and the supporting muscles of the abdomen.

Performance
1. With feet together, stand facing the *end* of the weight bench.
2. Step up with your right foot, standing erect on top of the bench.
3. Step down to the floor, starting with your left leg and trailing with your right.
4. Repeat the movement, stepping up with your left leg and continuing the sequence. That's a rep.
5. Continue to alternate legs until you've completed the required number of reps. That's a set.

Biomechanical Tips
Check your bench for stability before beginning this exercise. Spend the first workout without weights, perfecting your balance and practicing technique. Add 1 or 2 dumbbells after the technique has been mastered. In subsequent workouts, as the exercise movement becomes more coordinated, move to a barbell.

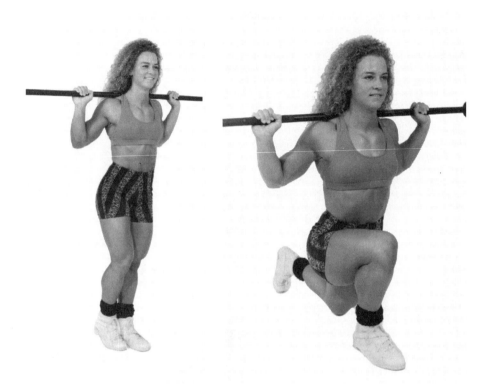

LUNGE

Muscles Involved

The quadriceps at the fronts of the thighs and the gluteal muscles of the buttocks, with secondary emphasis on the hamstrings, lower back, calves, and the supporting muscles of the abdomen.

Performance

1. Stand upright with feet placed shoulder width apart. Hold the barbell firmly on your shoulders.

2. Keeping head up and back straight, take a long step forward with either foot. Plant your foot and drop your hips until your lead thigh is parallel to the floor.

3. Push backward and upward with your lead foot until you are back at the starting position.

4. Repeat with the opposite leg. That's one rep.

Biomechanical Tips

Knee Care: Keeping your front heel on the ground helps keep your front knee above your foot as you drop into the low position.

The correct motion is a two-step procedure: First, step forward. Then, after stopping your forward motion, lower your body straight down into the low position by bending your knee.

Beginner's Tip

Spend the first several workouts practicing correct form *without using weights*. Once you're able to perfectly execute 10 reps with each leg without weight, add dumbbells or a barbell plate. Later, as balance continually improves, try a barbell if you wish.

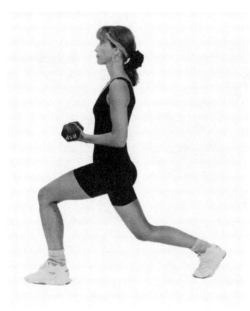

Variation:
Lunge with dumbbells

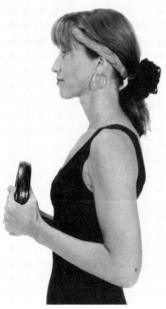

Variation:
Lunge with barbell plate

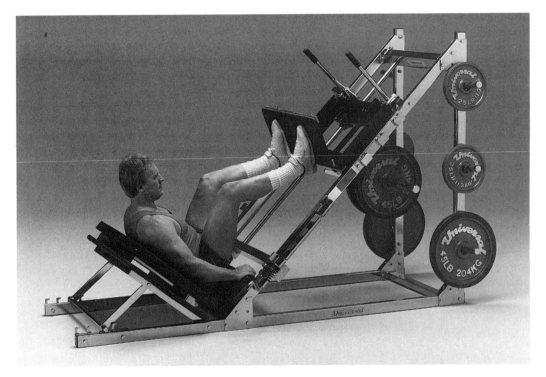

LEG PRESS

Muscles Involved

The quadriceps of the frontal thighs and gluteals of the buttocks with secondary emphasis on the hamstrings. Your arms and upper back will provide a supporting action.

Performance

1. Lie on backrest with feet on foot pad spaced 18' to 24' apart.
2. Press weight to the top position and release safety stops.
3. As you inhale, lower weight to the bottom position, knees bent at 90 to 110 degrees.
4. Holding your breath, press the weight to the top position.
5. Keep your hips down and your lower back pressed against the backrest during the entire movement.

Biomechanical Tip

Sometimes the tendons attaching the quadriceps to the tibia and fibula get sore from athletic competition. If you find that sore knees interfere with your leg presses, try moving your feet forward on the footpad of the machine (or the top pad of a horizontal-motion machine such as that found on a Universal multimachine).

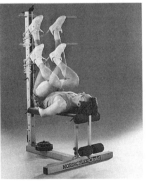

An inverted leg press exercise on a home unit

BASIC MOVEMENT TWO: PULL

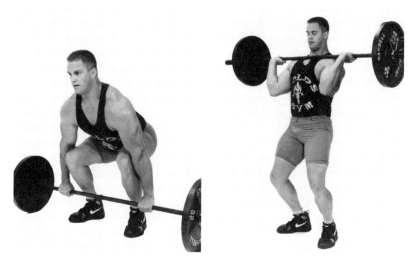

POWER CLEANS

Muscles Involved
All the back muscles, plus biceps, deltoids, forearms, thighs, gluteals, and calves.

Barbell Starting Position
Walk up to a barbell lying on the floor until your shins touch the bar. Place your feet about shoulder-width apart and point your toes slightly outward. Bend down and take a shoulder-width overhand grip on the bar, palms facing your shins, elbows straight. Bend your knees until your hips are above your knees but below your shoulders. Tense your spinal muscles to arch your back slightly. Look straight ahead. Keep facing forward throughout the movement.

Performance
1. In an explosive manner, start to straighten your legs to begin the barbell movement away from the floor. Be sure to keep your elbows straight at this point. They are only acting as cables to hook the barbell to your shoulders.
2. As your legs straighten, begin to extend your hips, keeping your elbows locked.

3. As your whole body reaches an erect posture, follow through on the pulling motion by rising on your toes and bending your elbows to swing the weight up to your shoulders.
4. To secure the barbell there, move your elbows under it and let the bar settle across your deltoids at the base of your neck.
5. Lower by reversing the above procedure (arms/hips/legs).
6. Repeat as required.

Biomechanical Tips
Always stick to this leg/hip/arms sequence when cleaning (pulling) a weight to your shoulders. Only by keeping your hips low and initiating the pull with your legs can you keep your lower back in the proper biomechanical position to minimize injuries. Also, with heavy weights, you will not be able to pull with arm strength if the bar has not already been accelerated by using the more powerful thighs and lower back. Remember to keep the movement explosive or you may have difficulty getting the barbell to your shoulders. Power cleans develop explosiveness and muscle-contraction speed for all athletic events.

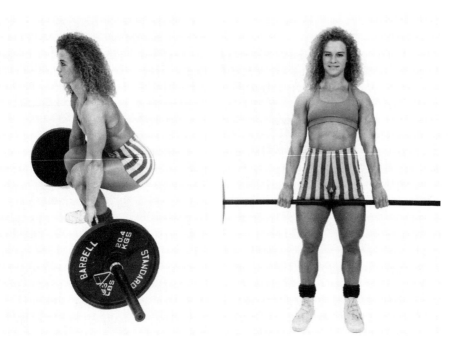

DEADLIFTS

Muscles Involved

The erector spinae and quadriceps, with secondary emphasis on the upper-back muscles, trapezius, forearms, hamstrings, and hip extensors. The abdominals and calves act as stabilizing muscles. Deadlifts are important to strengthen the muscles used to pull anything up from the ground, as in lifting a wrestling opponent from the mat.

Barbell Starting Position

Stand with your feet under the bar, shins resting against the bar. Your feet should be about shoulder-width apart, and your toes pointed slightly outward. Bend down and grasp the barbell handle with an overhand grip, your hands about shoulder width apart and your palms facing toward your shins. Bend your legs until your hips are below your shoulders and slightly above your knees. Arch your back by slightly tensing your lower-back muscles (erector spinae). Keep your head upright throughout the exercise and look straight ahead.

Performance

1. Pull the barbell up along your legs, first by straightening your legs and then extending at the hips to bring your body upright. When your body is completely straight and upright, the barbell will be resting across the tops of your thighs.

2. Lower the barbell slowly back along the same path, flexing at the hips first and then the legs as you return to the starting position.

3. Repeat as required.

Biomechanical Tips

It is vitally important to keep the leg straightening/hip extension sequence as you raise the weight and hip-flexing/leg-bending sequence as you lower the barbell. When straightening your legs to lift the weight, keep the bar as close to your body as possible. This minimizes the danger of lower-back straining.

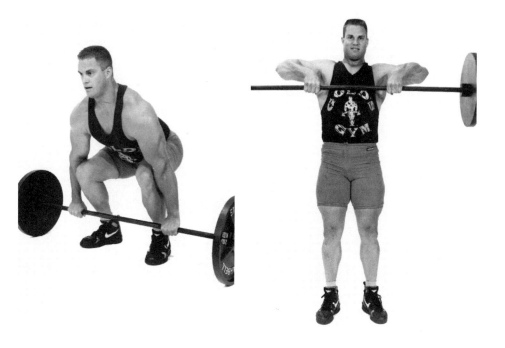

HIGH PULL

Muscles Involved
All of the back muscles, plus biceps, deltoids, forearms, thighs, gluteals, and calves.

Barbell Starting Position
Stand with your feet about 16" apart, shins touching the bar. Bend down and take an overhand grip on the bar. Bend your knees until your upper legs are parallel to the floor, your back is straight, and your eyes are looking forward.

Performance
1. Begin the exercise movement by straightening your legs, keeping your arms straight as the barbell rises from the floor.
2. As your legs straighten, your hips extend forward—initiating an erect posture. Your arms remain straight at this point of the exercise.
3. As your body reaches an erect posture, continue bringing the bar up by simultaneously pulling with the arms and rising on the toes until the bar reaches the highest possible point.
4. Control the bar by resisting the pull of gravity as the barbell is lowered to the floor. That's a rep.

Biomechanical Tips
Don't bounce the barbell between repetitions. Although bouncing is a temptation to initiate acceleration, each repetition should begin from a total stop with arms straight.

Mastering the leg/hip/arm sequence of the pull is the key to heavy power cleans. The powerful leg and lower-back muscles initiate the pull, accelerating the barbell so that the less-powerful muscles of the upper body can complete the movement.

Change the width of the hand spacing from workout to workout to more fully prepare the muscles for the variety of movements encountered in athletic competition.

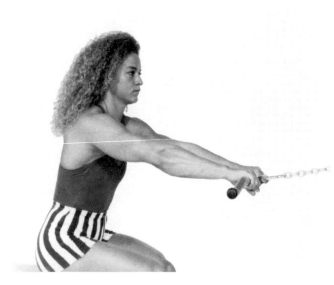 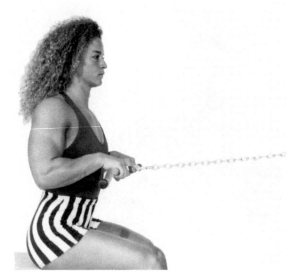

SEATED CABLE LONG PULL

Muscles Involved
All the back muscles, biceps, forearms, with secondary emphasis on quadriceps, hips, and gluteals.

Starting Position
Start the exercise with your torso at a 45-degree angle with the floor. Your arms, shoulders, and lats should be stretched forward to resist the pull of the weight.

Performance
1. Simultaneously straighten your torso until it is vertical to the floor while pulling with your arms until the pulley handle touches your rib cage. Your torso should be perpendicular to the floor, with your working shoulder rotated to the rear.
2. Return to the starting position, arms stretched forward and torso at a 45-degree angle with the floor. That's a rep.

Biomechanical Tips
Control the weight throughout the exercise movement. Don't accelerate the weight with a jerk at the beginning of the exercise or allow the momentum of the weight to overstretch your lower back at the end of the movement.

Training Tip
Handles and grips—the one-armed version of the long pull involves a rotation of the torso that does not occur with the more rigidly controlled two-armed version.

If you opt for two-armed long pulls, as illustrated, increase the variety of the movement by interchanging handles from workout to workout. Most gyms have a variety of bars and handles that can be attached to the cable machine.

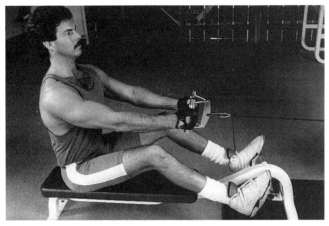

You can see from the picture of the Cybex® Low Pull
Station that the legs and lower back are integrally
involved in the long pull movement.

BASIC MOVEMENT THREE: KNEE LIFT

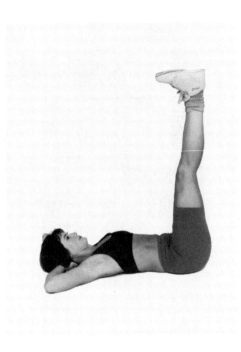

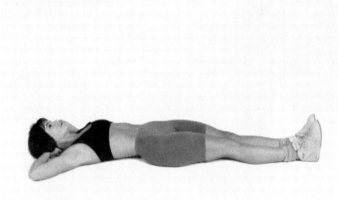

LEG RAISES

Muscles Involved
The frontal abdominals and the hip flexors (psoas and iliacus)

Starting Position
Lie on your back on the floor or on a sit-up board, with legs straight. Place your hands behind your head or under your hips.

Performance
1. Raise your legs straight up until they're perpendicular to the floor. Your feet will travel along an approximate 90-degree arc during the movement.
2. Lower your legs.
3. Repeat as required.

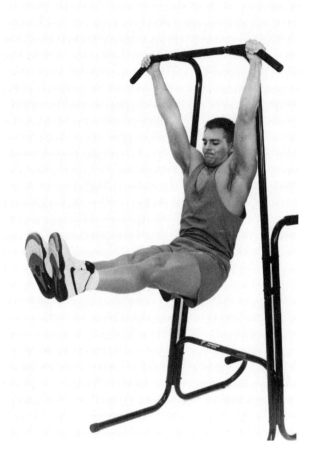

HANGING LEG RAISES

Muscles Involved

All of the frontal abdominal muscles and hip flexors (psoas and iliacus), with supporting assistance from the forearms.

Starting Position

Jump and grasp a chinning bar with an overhand grip, your hands about shoulder-width apart and your palms facing forward. Hang with your body straight below the bar and point your toes.

Performance

1. Keep your legs straight or bend them slightly at the knees.
2. Raise your legs until they are parallel to the floor. Throughout the movement keep your legs pressed together.
3. Lower to the initial position.
4. Repeat as required.

Biomechanical Tips

There is a tendency with this exercise for the body to begin swinging, which reduces the effectiveness of the movement. To keep from swinging, have a partner place his or her palm in the middle of your lower back to steady your body.

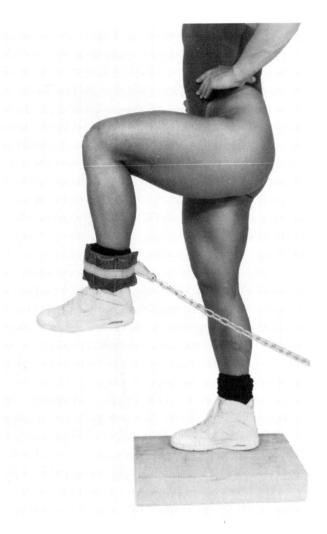

KNEE LIFT WITH PULLEY

Muscles Involved

The hip flexors with help from the lower abdominals.

Starting Position

Facing away from the low pulley machine, strap one ankle to the pulley cable. Hold a bench or bar for balance.

Performance

1. Lie on your back with both legs straight, one ankle strapped to a pulley cable. Brace the opposite foot to avoid sliding toward the pulley machine during the exercise.

2. Bend the knee of the leg attached to the cable, pulling it as far as possible toward your chest.

3. Under control, return your foot to the starting position. Repeat the required number of reps and switch legs.

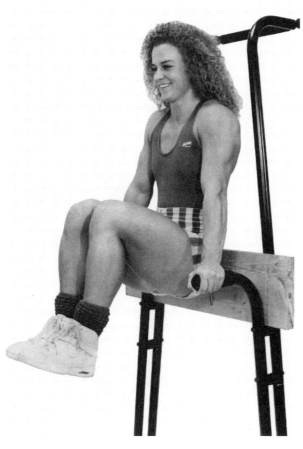 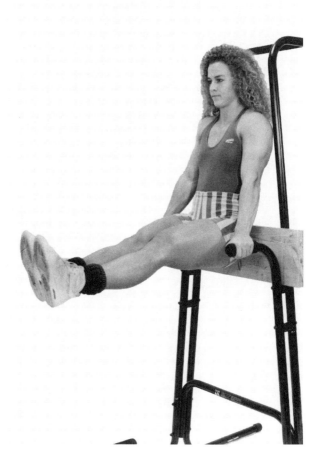

FROG KICKS

Muscles Involved

All of the frontal abdominals, the hip flexors (psoas and iliacus), and the gluteals, with supporting assistance from forearms.

Starting Position

At the starting point you will be supporting your body with straight arms on dip bars, knees pulled up and in as high as possible.

Performance

1. Keeping your legs together, extend your legs forward.
2. Return to the initial position.
3. Repeat as required.

Biomechanical Tips

To attack your hip flexors and abdominals from slightly different angles, spread your legs different distances apart as you pull in and extend your knees. Each leg position will hit the abdominals a little differently, and the accumulation of all possible positions will result in super-knee-lift strength.

BASIC MOVEMENT FOUR: TRUNK ROTATION

REVERSE TRUNK TWIST

Muscles Involved
The abdominals, obliques, and lower back.

Starting Position
Lie on your back on the floor, arms extended to your sides, knees bent, thighs vertical to the floor.

Performance
1. Slowly lower your knees to one side of your body, keeping the thighs perpendicular to your torso as you touch the floor.
2. Return to the knee-vertical start position and lower your thighs to the opposite side.
3. Return to vertical. That's a rep.

Biomechanical Tips
The reverse trunk twist is the most basic of the exercises available to strengthen the muscles responsible for the rotation of the torso.

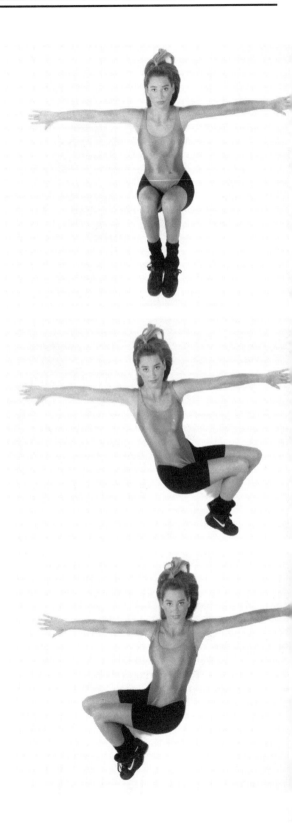

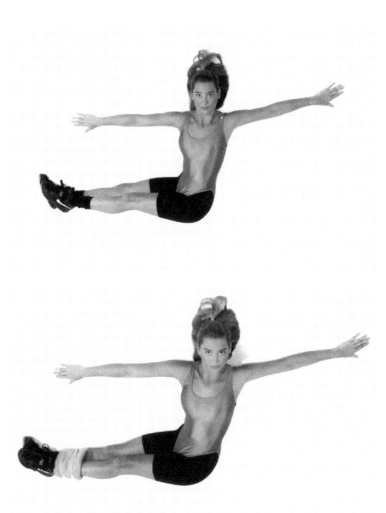

Variation: Reverse trunk twist—straight legs with ankle weight
As your ability to perform the exercise improves, the resistance can be increased sequentially by (1) straightening the legs and (2) adding ankle weights.

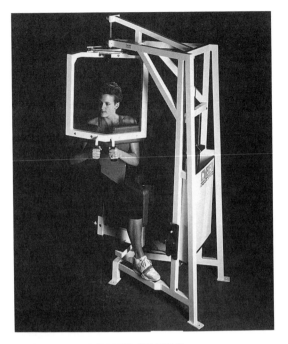

CYBEX® ROTARY TORSO

Muscles Involved
The internal and external obliques, deep posterior rotators, longissimus, iliocostalis.

Performance
1. Adjust seat height so that upper pads are positioned across your shoulders.

2. Place your legs securely against the adductor pads and select a comfortable foot position.

3. Release upper pullbutton and move machine arm to desired start position. The start position is adjustable in 15-degree increments.

4. Maintain contact with chest pad and grasp handles.

5. Rotate your torso slowly through the desired range of motion.

6. Slowly return to the start position with a smooth, controlled motion.

7. Move pullbutton to start position on opposite side and repeat the exercise for other side of torso.

Biomechanical Tip
This rotary torso machine offers an effective combination of upper- and lower-body stabilization to fully isolate torso muscles and to promote proper axis alignment.

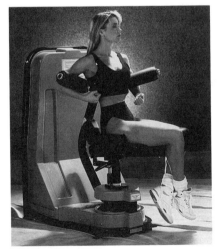

Variation: Nautilus® Rotary Torso

BASIC MOVEMENT FIVE: PUSH

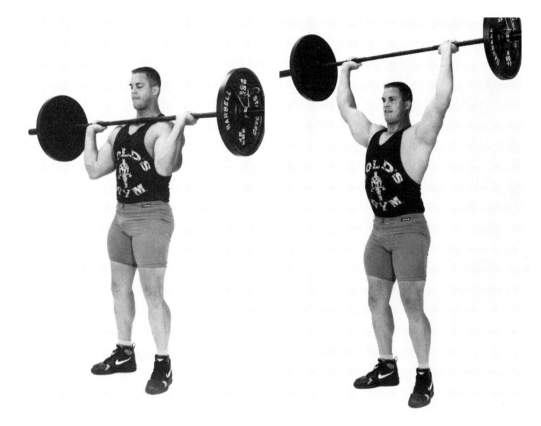

BARBELL PUSH PRESS

Muscles Involved

The deltoids of your shoulders and the triceps on the backs of your upper arms, with secondary emphasis on the upper pectorals, trapezius, lower back, and abdominals.

Barbell Starting Position

Bring the barbell to your shoulders so that it rests in front of your neck and across your shoulders. Your knees are slightly bent.

Performance

1. Straightening your legs explosively, push the barbell straight up past your face until your elbows are locked straight and the weight is directly over your head.

2. Bend your elbows to return the weight to your shoulders.

3. Repeat.

4. Once you have performed the required number of repetitions, return the barbell to the floor by bending first your legs and then flexing your hips as you lower it.

Biomechanical Tips

Minimize bending backward as you press the bar up. Excessive bending action will make the bar go up easier, but it will also put an unnecessary strain on your lower back. Be sure, as well, that the bar doesn't hit your nose on the way up.

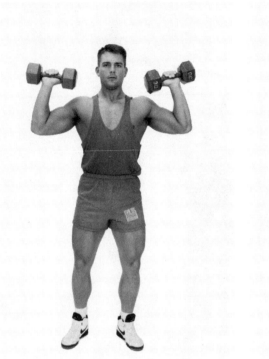
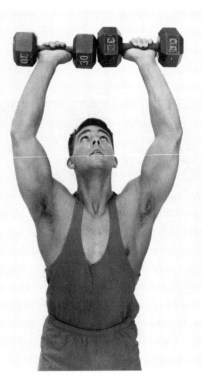

DUMBBELL PUSH PRESS

Muscles Involved

The deltoids and triceps, with secondary emphasis on the upper pectoral, trapezius, and legs. The lower back and abdominals act as stabilizers.

Starting Position

Stand erect, your feet shoulder-width apart, knees slightly bent, and your toes pointed outward slightly, a dumbbell in each hand, either resting on or positioned off your shoulders. Your palms should be facing forward at your shoulders, the same as for a barbell push press.

Performance

1. Using the acceleration from straightening your legs, push the dumbbells straight up to arm's length overhead, the two inner plates together.

2. Bend your elbows and return the dumbbells to the starting position.

3. Repeat as required.

Biomechanical Tips

The primary advantages of pressing dumbbells in place of a barbell are greater range of motion and the possibility of varied hand positions. With dumbbells, you can lower your hands below the level of your shoulders, while the barbell would run into your shoulder muscles before your hands could be lowered to the full possible extent of the pressing range of motion. Besides facing your palms forward when you press dumbbells, you can try facing them toward each other or at any other angle you desire.

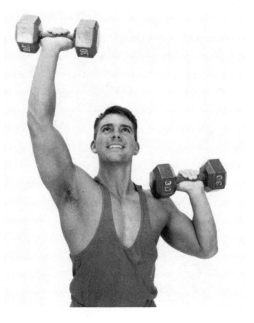

ALTERNATE DUMBBELL PUSH PRESS

Muscles Involved
The deltoids and triceps, with secondary emphasis on the upper pectoral, trapezius, and legs. The lower back and abdominals act as stabilizers.

Starting Position
Stand erect, your feet shoulder-width apart, knees slightly bent, and your toes pointed outward slightly, a dumbbell in each hand, either resting on or positioned off your shoulders. Your palms should be facing forward, at your shoulders, the same as for a barbell push press.

Performance
1. Using the acceleration from straightening your legs, push one dumbbell straight up to arm's length overhead.
2. Bend your elbow and return the dumbbell to the starting position.
3. Alternate to the other dumbbell and duplicate movement.
4. Repeat as required.

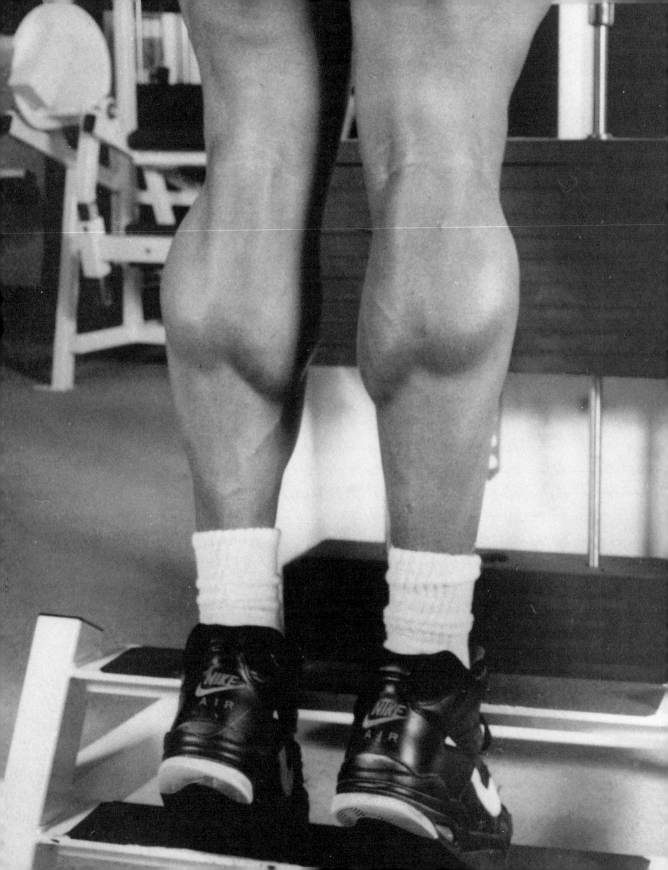

Establishing Training Priorities: Modifying Your Exercise Program

The portion of your total training time devoted to strength training depends on your sport.

Power athletes, such as throwers and football players, so heavily depend on strength training that the weight room becomes a second home. Endurance athletes, marathoners, and distance swimmers waste little time building bulging biceps. Instead they spend the majority of total training time—and energy—running or swimming mile after mile.

Whatever the relative importance of strength training to your athletic success, maximizing training time in the weight room requires establishing training priorities. Three factors continually impact training priorities:

1. Exercise selection
2. Modifying standard exercises to copy specific sports movements
3. Selective size gains

The following material will help you design a personal, success-oriented, strength-training program that maximizes your training time.

SELECTING THE BEST EXERCISE

There are thousands of strength-training exercises, including the ones in this book. Your immediate goal is to select the handful of exercises that best strengthen the movements of your sport.

Exercise selection is a 4-step process:

1. Identify a competition movement that you want to strengthen.
2. Identify the Basic Movement that is closest to the competitive movement.
3. Explore the group of exercises that strengthen the Basic Movement in question.
4. Select the one exercise from the group that most closely duplicates the competition movement.

Let's use a high jumper as a quick study of the selection process. The first step is to *identify the movement* needing strengthening. For the high jumper, straightening the knee of the takeoff leg is the best example.

The second step is to *identify the Basic Movement* responsible for the movement. Leg Drive is the obvious choice.

The third step is to *explore the group of exercises* that strengthen leg drive. There are several exercises in that group (see pages 92 to 98). But for the sake of brevity, we'll narrow the choice to the squat and step-up.

The final step is to *select the one exercise* from the appropriate group that most closely duplicates the actual sports movement, straightening the knee of the takeoff leg in the case of our high jumper. Both the squat and step-up straighten the knee, but the exercise that most closely duplicates the jumper's competition movement is the step-up, so the step-up is the right exercise for a high jumper to perform.

There are many other movements that the high jumper wants to strengthen: the knee lift of the lead leg, the arm and shoulder drive at takeoff, and so on. The appropriate exercises to strengthen each of those movements are selected through the same 4-step process.

· Identifying the Muscle Group Responsible for the Movement

Muscles propel movements. Knowing which muscles propel which movements is helpful in understanding the rationale for exercise selection. The following illustrations will help you identify the major muscle groups responsible for your general sports movements. For each labeled group, the commonly used name of the muscle is listed, followed when necessary by the scientific name.

Throughout the book, exercise descriptions are accompanied by a description of the responsible muscle groups. But remember that strength training for sports is movement driven: don't get trapped into a mind-set of "training muscles." Select the strength training exercise that most closely duplicates the movement of your sport.

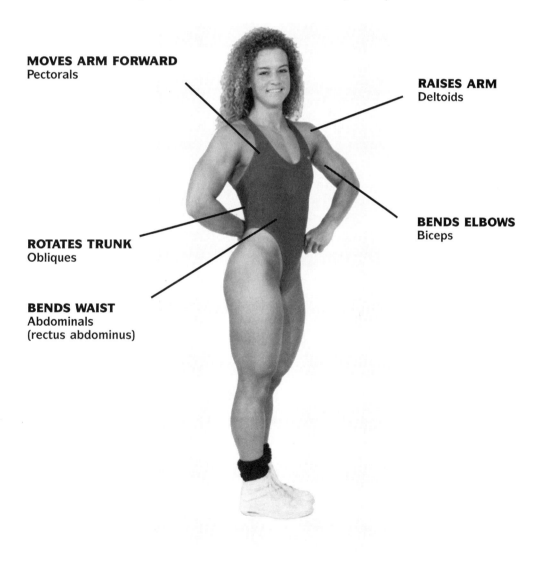

MOVES ARM FORWARD
Pectorals

RAISES ARM
Deltoids

BENDS ELBOWS
Biceps

ROTATES TRUNK
Obliques

BENDS WAIST
Abdominals
(rectus abdominus)

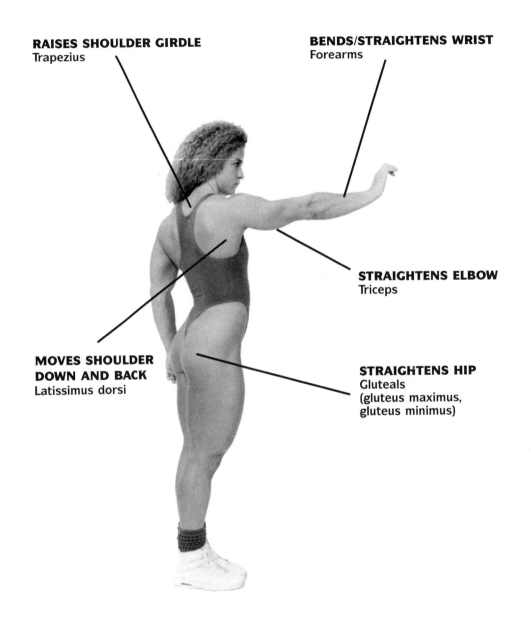

RAISES SHOULDER GIRDLE
Trapezius

BENDS/STRAIGHTENS WRIST
Forearms

STRAIGHTENS ELBOW
Triceps

**MOVES SHOULDER
DOWN AND BACK**
Latissimus dorsi

STRAIGHTENS HIP
Gluteals
(gluteus maximus,
gluteus minimus)

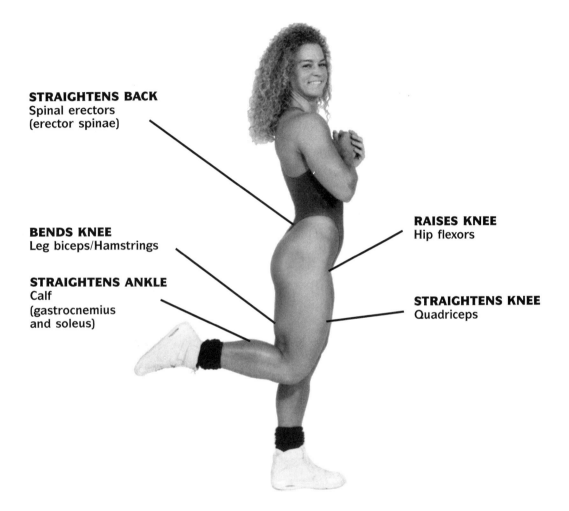

STRAIGHTENS BACK
Spinal erectors
(erector spinae)

BENDS KNEE
Leg biceps/Hamstrings

STRAIGHTENS ANKLE
Calf
(gastrocnemius
and soleus)

RAISES KNEE
Hip flexors

STRAIGHTENS KNEE
Quadriceps

· A Practical Method of Identifying Muscles Responsible for Movements

One method of identifying the primary movements and muscles of your sport—the movements and muscles most needing strengthening—is identifying what's sore after an especially heavy sports workout or after that first training session following a layoff. Because the muscles used the most will become the sorest, this method can identify the key muscle groups and movements contributing to your sport.

MODIFYING STANDARD EXERCISES TO COPY YOUR SPORTS MOVEMENTS

Standard strength-training exercises—the Basic and Isolated Movements in this book—can be modified to more closely approximate your sports movement by changing the grip, limb orientation, or the recommended form.

The closer the exercise copies the sports movement, the more likely that the increased strength will transfer to the playing field.

You may actually use less weight for the modified movement. That's okay. Your primary concern is to build strength that can be applied to competition movements, not strength that is useful only in the gym. Choose the modification that best duplicates your sports movement, then select an appropriate weight.

· Modify Grips and Attachments

Grips contribute to limb orientation, and limb orientation during strength training determines the precise movement (and muscles) that will be strengthened.

There is a variety of handgrips and attachments available for use with many pieces of weight training equipment. The greatest variety is often located with the pulley equipment found in most commercial gyms.

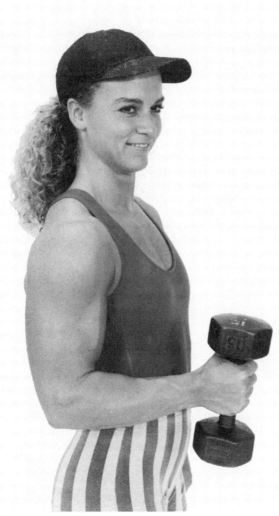

Hammer curl

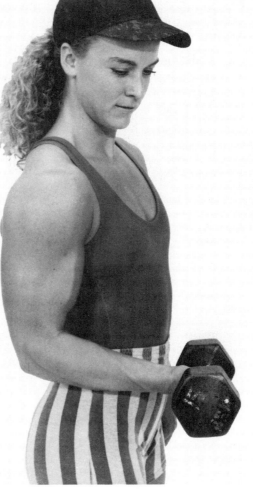

Regular dumbbell curl You can demonstrate the importance of choosing the right grip by curling a dumbbell with two different grip positions, an underhand grip and a knuckles-out grip, as illustrated. Each places a markedly different stress on your biceps and forearm.

· **Modify Limb and Torso Orientation**

While grip determines limb orientation some of the time, constant attention should be directed toward matching limb orientation during the strength exercise with that of the sports movement.

Let's use the example of two variations of the bench press, regular and close-grip, as they apply to the discus thrower. A discus thrower would benefit most from regular bench presses (see page 158): the elbow is kept away from the torso, as is the case during the discus throw. The close-grip bench press is performed with the elbows kept close to the torso. The orientation of the upper arm during the regular bench press more closely matches the throwing motion.

As you exercise, constantly monitor the orientation of your legs, arms, torso, feet, knees—all your joint-related positions—to make sure you're actually strengthening the precise movement of your sport.

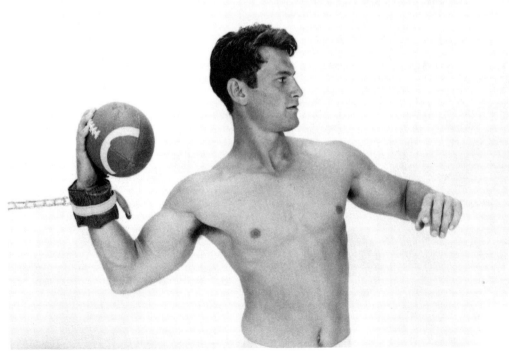

Football cable

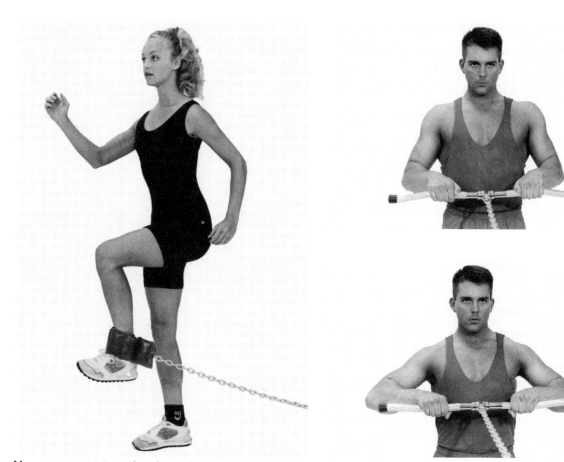

You may want to take the grip one step further by attaching a cable to a sports implement—or your wrist or ankle—to more closely mimic the athletic movement of your choice.

Elbow out The long pull offers a graphic example that differentiates grip from limb orientation. The orientation of the upper arm can be positioned through numerous angles while the handgrip remains the same.

· Modify "Strict" Form?

Strict form refers to duplicating exercise technique according to instructions, but much of what I've said so far suggests doing just the opposite. That's because traditional exercise technique is often wrong for the athlete.

For decades, bodybuilders and bodybuilding magazines have been the technical journals for weight training exercises. It's important that you don't compare your exercise form—or exercise selection and program design, for that matter—with a bodybuilder's.

Bodybuilders follow a different protocol, focusing on building muscle to change appearance rather than to increase movement strength.

The concept of strict form in the weight room originated with bodybuilders wanting to isolate specific muscle groups or muscles within a group. The isolation of specific muscles doesn't work for athletes because competition, and therefore the goal of training movements, requires the synchronous movement of many muscle groups required during athletic competition.

This is not to say that strictly following recommended technique isn't important for safety. There are exercises where the recommended form should be strictly followed. But when form is not a safety factor, recommendations on form should be seen as suggestions rather than rules.

Exercise machines create another obstacle for athletes wanting to vary the recommended lifting technique in order to better duplicate a sports movement. In order to sell the greatest number of machines, manufacturers design them for the generalist, someone wanting general strength or appearance changes in a given muscle group and who's willing to be bound by the machine's controlled movement.

Though it's more of a problem than modifying free-weight exercise, a little ingenuity goes a long way when changing machine movements to meet specific athletic needs. For example, the single-leg leg press shown opposite is much more likely to benefit the athlete than the traditional two-leg version. The athlete rarely drives simultaneously off both legs during competition, instead relying on a single supporting leg. Using one limb rather than two during a machine exercise can enhance coordination and synergy among the secondary muscle groups that contribute to that movement.

Regardless of exercise equipment, the important point to remember is: Don't choose limb orientation because of convenience or the ability to lift heavier weights; duplicate the limb orientation of your sports movement.

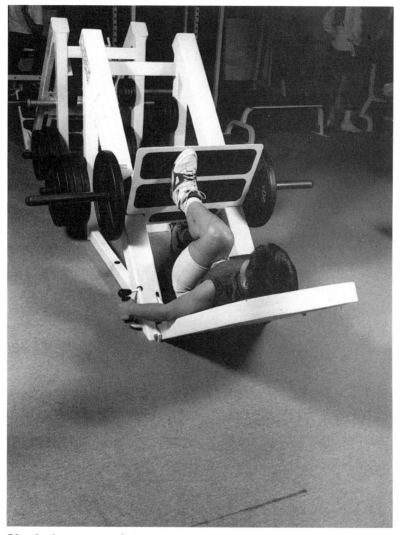

Single-leg press Substitute single-leg presses for the standard double-leg press during alternate workouts. The training effect is markedly different. On the inverted leg-press machine, cheat your body to one side of the backrest so that your foot is positioned at the center of the footpad.

SELECTIVE SIZE GAINS

Increased strength is universally desirable in athletics, but increasing the size of the body—even the size of the muscles—can be a detriment.

You can increase the strength of a muscle, to a point, without increasing the size of a muscle. That is possible because of the so-called neural adaptations discussed in chapter 2. But strength gains beyond neural adaptations are accompanied by an increase in size. For your athletic success, limit that increase in size to the muscles directly contributing to your event.

Selective size gains go hand-in-hand with the selection and prioritization of exercises:

1. Limit exercise selection to those that directly contribute to strengthening the technical movements of your sport. That way, any size gains will be muscle that contributes to your athletic movements.

2. Adjust the training intensity for these exercises to reflect their importance. For example, do 3 sets of one exercise but only 2 of another, depending on the relative contribution of the exercise.

Bigger, stronger muscles must more than carry their own weight or all the effort and energy building them has been a waste of time. That's the case whether the athlete is a hulking football player smashing opposing linemen or the slender high jumper fighting gravity. The additional muscle must generate additional power that can be incorporated into the athletic movement.

The problem comes when you've increased the size of nonfunctional muscle, muscle not contributing to the event technique. For example, increasing the size of the high jumper's chest, shoulders, and arms adds useless body weight, a handicap when elevating the body over the bar.

The analogy of the high jumper holds for all athletes. Unnecessary size is a handicap to the working muscles and your overall performance. That's why selective size gains are of the utmost importance to the serious athlete.

• • •

The time has come for you to adapt your Basic Movement Program. Select from the exercises in this book, mofifying where necessary, or move beyond the book and develop your own exercises, always thinking "safety" as you refer to the suggestions throughout this and other chapters.

NAME			WORKOUT		CHART	
	DATE	WEIGHT	SETS	REPS	Notes	Comments
LEG DRIVE						
PULL						
KNEE LIFT						
TRUNK ROTATION						
PUSH						
SPECIALTY EXERCISES*						

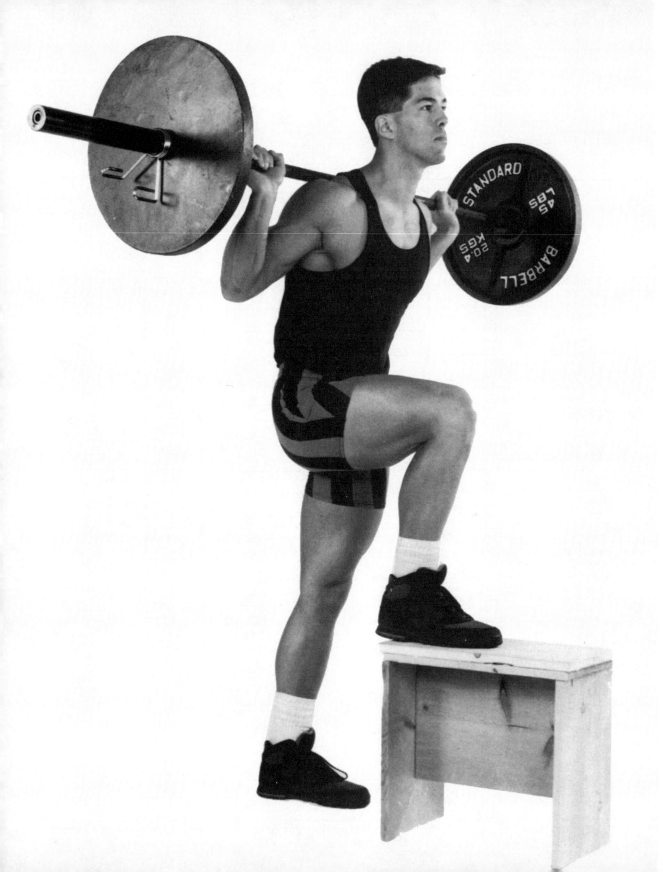

9
Isolation Exercises: Small Parts of Larger Movements

The Basic Movements, described in chapter 7, can be broken down into smaller segments called isolated movements. This chapter is devoted to the exercises that strengthen those smaller, isolated movements.

To illustrate the concept, squat for several reps as you're reading this passage. Your squatting demonstrates Leg Drive, one of the five Basic Movements. Close examination of your Leg Drive (squat) reveals that 3 joints—the hip, knee, and ankle—straighten during the upside of the movement. The straightening of each joint—included in the larger, more dynamic Basic Movement—is an example of Isolated Movements.

There are exercises for strengthening each of these Isolated Movements. For example, leg extensions (page 136) strengthen the straightening of the knee, calf raises (pages 134, 137, 138) strengthen the straightening of the ankle, and the stiff-legged deadlift (page 100) strengthens the straightening of the hips. In combination, the three exercises strengthen the larger Basic Movement. The parts equal the whole.

WHY PRACTICE ISOLATION EXERCISES?

Four of the many reasons you might include isolation exercises into your program are:
- to rehabilitate injuries surrounding a particular joint
- to correct a "weak link" in a Basic Movement
- to prevent injury by strengthening a body part that endures disproportionate competitive stress
- to add to the Basic Movement Program, strengthening small, technical movements that aren't sufficiently strengthened with Basic Movement exercises

RECOMMENDED USE OF ISOLATION EXERCISES

Isolation exercises play an important part in strength training. Their primary impact, as noted above, is to strengthen important competitive movements that are undertrained if relying exclusively on the Basic Movement Program.

In chapter 10 there are almost 30 different strength training programs for more than 30 different sports. That's because each sport and athlete has different strength needs. *Isolation exercises are recommended as part of each and every Packaged Program.* They are recommended to meet identifiable strength needs not met by the Basic Program.

If you are designing your own strength program with (or without) the help of chapter 8, I recommend that you seriously consider isolated exercises. Particularly, as outlined above, for rehabilitation, correcting a weak link, injury prevention, and strengthening a movement not adequately strengthened with the Basic Movement Program.

That is not to say that the Basic Movement Program should be overridden. It is the foundation of your strength training program; isolated movements are additions, not substitutions.

ISOLATION EXERCISE DESCRIPTIONS

In this chapter the isolation exercises have been listed according to the Basic Movement to which they belong. The following chart details the groupings:

	Free-Weight Exercise	**Machine Exercise**
Leg Drive		
	Partial squats	
	Barbell seated calf raise	Leg-extension machine
	Seated calf raise with weight	
	Donkey calf raise	
	One-legged calf raise	
Pull		
	Chin-ups	Lat-machine pulldown
	Bent row with barbell	
	Bent row with dumbbell	Bent row machine
	Upright row with barbell	Cable upright row
	Stiff-legged deadlift	
	Good mornings	
	Hyperextensions	Back-extension machine
	Bent-arm pullovers	Pullover machine
	Straight-arm pullovers	
	Side lateral raises	
	Seated side lateral raises	
	Barbell biceps curls	Biceps curl machine
	Reverse barbell curls	
	Dumbbell curls	Pulley curls
	Concentration curls	Nautilus® curl
Trunk Rotation		
	Sit-ups	Home unit sit-ups
	Decline sit-ups with weight	Universal® Abdominal Machine

	Free-Weight Exercise	**Machine Exercise**
Push	Bench press	Universal® DVR Bench Press
		Cybex® Chest Press
	Dumbbell bench press	
	Close grip bench press	
	Incline bench press	
	Incline bench dumbbell press	
	Chest fly on flat or incline bench	Cybex® Fly Machine
		Universal® Vertical Chest Bench
	Press behind the neck	
	Seated press behind the neck	Soloflex® behind-the-neck press
	Dips	
	Lying barbell triceps extensions	
	Standing barbell triceps extensions	Nautilus® Triceps Extensions
	Dumbbell triceps extensions	
	Single-Arm dumbbell triceps extensions	
Specialty Exercises	Dumbbell wrist curls	Nautilus® 4-Way Neck Machine
	Barbell wrist curls	Cybex® Seated Leg Curl
	Rotator cuff series	Nordic® Standing Leg Curl

LEG DRIVE: ISOLATION EXERCISES

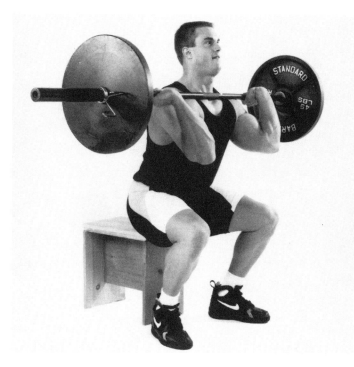

PARTIAL SQUATS

Muscles Involved
The quadriceps of the frontal thigh and gluteal muscles of the buttocks, with secondary emphasis on the hamstrings, lower back, and supporting muscles of the abdominals.

Barbell Starting Position
Because you will be doing less-than-full repetitions of the squat, the starting position for partial squats is the same as for full squats.

Performance
There are 4 common types of partial squats—quarter squats (one-fourth of the way down), half squats, three-quarter squats, and bench squats (as illustrated). Bench squats are done to a depth at which your buttocks touch a bench that you are straddling while doing the movement. Other than the depth, partial squats are performed exactly like full squats.

Biomechanical Tips
Because you will be able to use significantly more weight for partial squats than for full squats, it will be a good idea to concentrate on keeping your back muscles under tension throughout the movement. This will prevent you from relaxing at any point in the movement, which can leave your lower back vulnerable to injury. Keeping your back muscles tensed is vital when doing bench squats because there is a natural tendency to sit on the bench for a moment at the bottom of each repetition. To prevent this, try to just "touch" the bench before starting up. Never, however, bounce on the bench when doing bench squats. For all squatting movements, you can also use a weight-lifting belt (more on this later) to give added support to your abdomen and lumbar muscles.

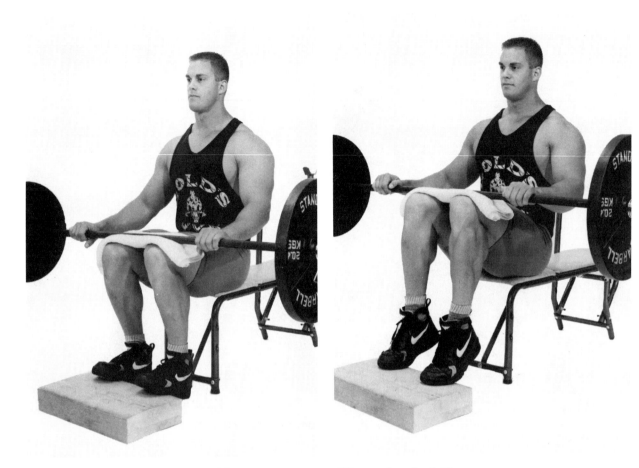

BARBELL SEATED CALF RAISE

Muscles Involved
The soleus muscle of the calf, with significant emphasis on the gastrocnemius.

Starting Position
Sit down on a bench with your toes on the footboard and a barbell across the tops of your knees.

Performance
1. Rise up and down on your toes with the resistance provided by the barbell.
2. To secure the weight at the completion of a set, simply move the barbell to the floor.

Biomechanical Tips
The broad soleus muscle under the gastrocnemius is fully contracted and stimulated only when you rise on your toes with a bent leg, so this is one of the few exercises in which you can do meaningful work for the soleus. As a variation, you can place a barbell plate across your knees to perform this exercise.

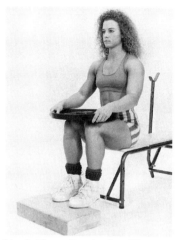

Variation: Seated calf raise with barbell plate

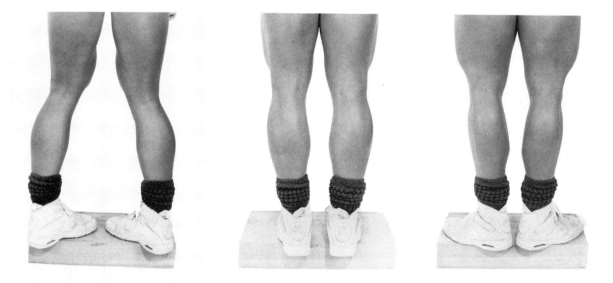

Vary Your Foot Position

Alternate foot positions occasionally, doing some sets with your feet parallel, some with toes pointed out at a 45-degree angle, and others with the toes pointed in at 45 degrees. Using all three toe positions will build more complete strength in the quadriceps.

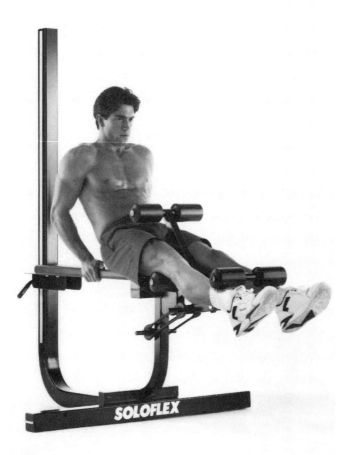

LEG EXTENSION

Muscles Involved

Almost totally the quadriceps, with a minimum of support from the arms, abdominals, and both upper and lower back. Quadriceps strength is helpful in any movement during which you extend your legs from a partially or fully bent position, such as running or jumping.

Starting Position

Sit on the edge of a free-weight leg-extension machine and hook the tops of your feet under the lower set of rollers. Steady your upper body by grasping the sides of the bench beside your hips.

Performance

1. Fully extend your legs with quadriceps strength until your knees lock.
2. Pause in the top position for one count.
3. Lower to the starting position.
4. Repeat as required.

Biomechanical Tips

Alternate foot position occasionally, doing some sets with your feet parallel, some with toes pointed out at a 45-degree angle, and others with the toes pointed in at 45 degrees. Using all three toe positions will build more complete strength in your quadriceps.

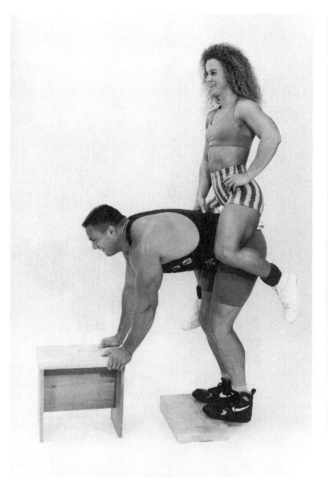 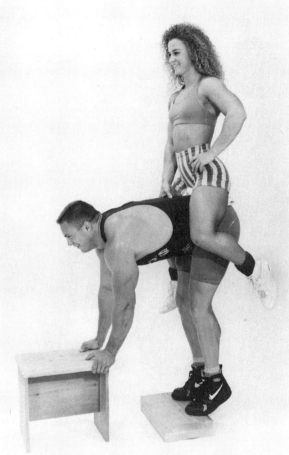

DONKEY CALF RAISES

Muscles Involved
Calf muscles, soleus, and gastrocnemius.

Starting Position
Bend over a flat bench from your waist until your torso is parallel to the floor and steady your torso by placing your hands—elbows locked—on the bench. Stand with your toes on a wooden block or at the edge of a raised platform on which the bench is placed. Have a partner jump up astride your hips, as if you were a horse, to provide resistance.

Performance
Rise up and down on your toes to stimulate your calves.

Biomechanical Tips
The heavier your partner, the more resistance provided, but it is necessary that he or she always sit in the same place on your back. Try to have your partner sit back as far as possible without falling off, because he or she will provide more resistance that way.

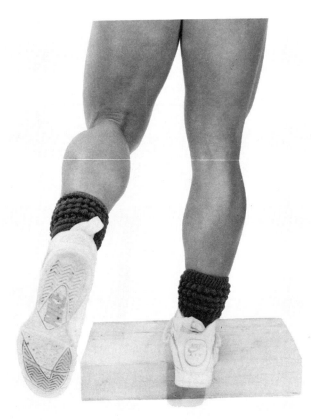

ONE-LEGGED CALF RAISE

Muscles Involved
Calf muscles, soleus, and gastrocnemius.

Dumbbell Starting Position
Put one foot on a block and slide your heel out away from the block until only the ball of your foot is in contact with the block. Hold a light dumbbell in one hand on the same side as the foot in contact with the block, your arm hanging straight down at your side, your palm facing the side of your body. Balance yourself by grasping an upright post or bar with your free hand.

Performance
1. Rise up and down on the toes of one foot to stimulate your calf.
2. Switch feet for the next set.
3. Count a full group of repetitions for both legs as a full set.

Biomechanical Tips
By concentrating your attention on one leg at a time, you will often be able to obtain a better calf workout.

PULL: ISOLATION EXERCISES

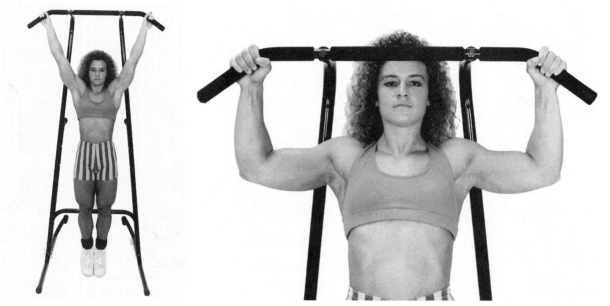

CHIN-UPS

Muscles Involved
The latissimus dorsi and biceps, with secondary emphasis on the deltoids and forearms.

Chinning Bar Starting Position
Grasp a horizontal bar with your hands at shoulder-width or wider, palms facing away from your body. At the start of a chin-up, you will be hanging straight down from the bar or hanging with your knees bent so that your thighs and calves form a 45-degree angle.

Performance
1. Consciously stretch your latissimus and then pull your body up until your upper arms are parallel with the bar. Keep your legs bent as you bring your body up. Be sure to arch your back and force your elbows down and back at the top of the movement.
2. Lower to initial position.
3. Repeat as required.

Biomechanical Tips
By varying the width of your grip, or by pulling up to the bar behind your neck, you can hit the upper back from numerous subtly different angles. By doing as many variations as possible, you will develop the best quality of pulling strength.

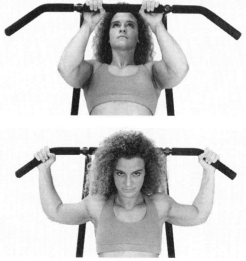

Variation: chin-ups

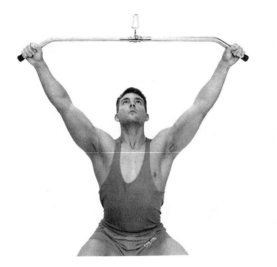

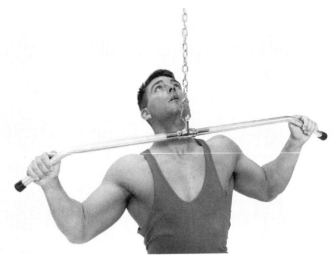

LAT MACHINE PULLDOWNS

Muscles Involved

The latissimus dorsi, with secondary emphasis on the biceps, forearms, and posterior deltoids.

Lat Machine Starting Position

Sit down at the lat-machine pulldown station, facing the weight stack. Grasp the handles at the ends of the lat pulley bar with each hand 6 to 12 inches beyond shoulder width. Your palms should be facing forward, away from your body.

Performance

1. Pull the bar down until it touches the base of your neck behind your head.

2. Return to the starting position, arms straight, and pull the next rep to the front of your neck.

3. Alternate pulling to back and front as required.

Biomechanical Tips

Kinesiologists tell us that the function of the latissimus dorsi is to pull the upper arms down and back, so emphasize pulling your elbows down and back on each repetition. Occasionally vary the grips—from wide to narrow, underhand or behind the neck—for more complete strength development.

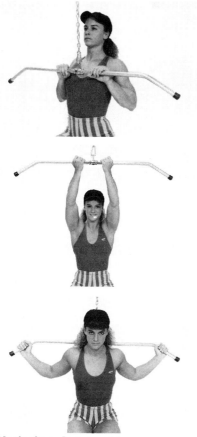

**Variation: Lat machine
pull-down grips**

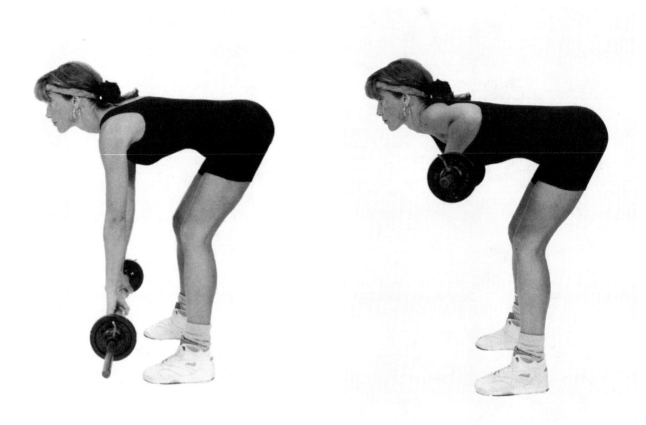

BENT ROW WITH BARBELL

Muscles Involved

The latissimus dorsi of the upper back, with secondary emphasis on biceps, trapezius, erector spinae, and forearm muscles.

Barbell Starting Position

Bend over until your torso is parallel to the floor. Your feet should be about shoulder-width apart, with toes pointed out slightly. Your arms should be hanging straight down. In this position, grasp a barbell with an overhand grip, your hands shoulder-width apart and your palms facing your shins. Bend your knees slightly.

Performance

1. Pull the barbell up until it touches your lower rib cage.
2. Lower the barbell slowly to the starting point.
3. Repeat.

Biomechanical Tips

Your upper arms should be moved to a 45-degree angle from your torso as the barbell is pulled upward. This results in the most favorable biomechanical position for maximum upper-back stimulation. To prevent lower-back-muscle injuries, keep your knees unlocked, and tense your spinal muscles enough to bring your spine into a slightly arched position.

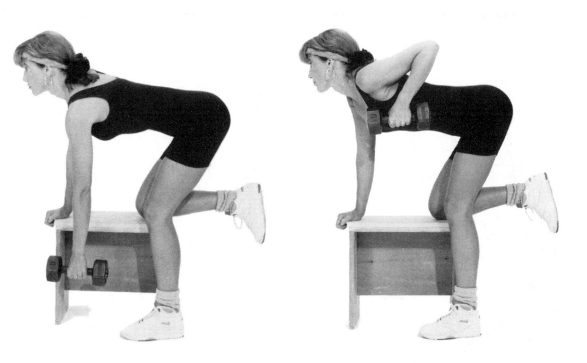

BENT ROW WITH DUMBBELL

Muscles Involved
The latissimus dorsi of the upper back, with secondary emphasis on biceps, trapezius, erector spinae, and forearm muscles.

Starting Position
Position your right knee and right hand on the bench; keep your back straight and parallel with the floor. The dumbbell hangs from your left arm.

Performance
1. Point your elbow toward the ceiling as you pull the dumbbell to your shoulder.
2. Lower the dumbbell toward the floor, fully stretching your upper back, shoulder, and arm at the low position.
3. After completing a set, switch positions and repeat the exercise for the right side.

Biomechanical Tip
Working with dumbbells rather than a barbell increases the range of motion, building a greater strength range for athletic movements.

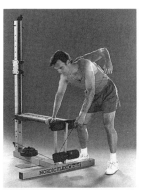

Variation: An equivalent exercise can be done with cable as demonstrated on this Nordic Flex Gold® home unit.

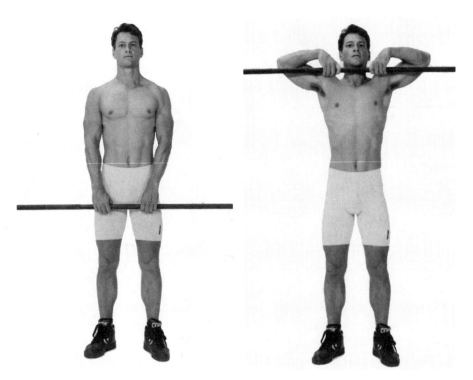

UPRIGHT ROW

Muscles Involved

The trapezius, with secondary emphasis on deltoids, biceps, and forearms.

Barbell Starting Position

Stand erect with your feet about shoulder-width apart and your toes pointed slightly outward. Take a 6-to-12-inch-wide overhand grip on the middle of a barbell handle and hold the barbell across your upper thighs with straight arms. Your palms should face your body.

Performance

1. Pull the bar up your body to your chin, emphasizing an elbows-up position at the top of the movement. Keep the barbell close to your body throughout the movement and sag your shoulders down at the beginning of each repetition.
2. Lower slowly.
3. Repeat as required.

Biomechanical Tips

It is important to tense the upper-back muscles at the top of the movement by forcing your shoulders back. Keep your lower-back muscles tight throughout the movement to prevent lumbar injuries.

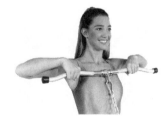

Variation: Cable Upright Row

If using a pulley-machine unit, use the low pulley station and grasp the pulley handle with your hands 6 inches apart and the handle resting across the tops of your thighs, palms facing your thighs.

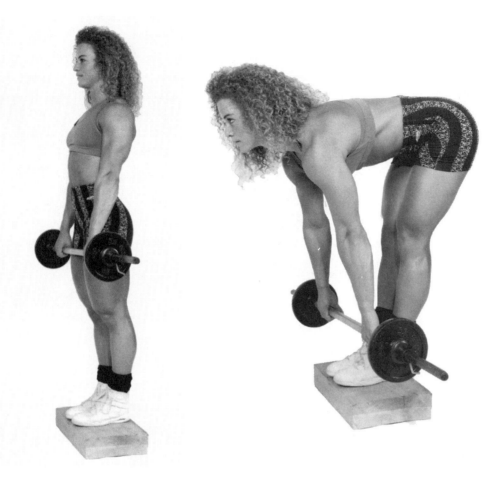

STIFF-LEGGED DEADLIFT

Muscles Involved
The lower back (spinal erectors), with secondary emphasis on the hamstrings, upper back, buttocks, and forearms.

Barbell Starting Position
Stand erect with your feet together and your toes pointed forward. Take an overhand grip on a barbell, palms facing your body, hands shoulder-width apart. Rest the barbell across the tops of your thighs with your arms straight.

Performance
1. Keeping your knees locked, bend slowly forward at the waist as far as possible.
2. Return to the upright position.
3. Repeat as required.

Biomechanical Tips
Because lifting with legs straight puts the back in a bad biomechanical position, it is vital to do the reps slowly to avoid lower-back strain. And because the barbell plates will touch the floor and keep the range of movement short, try standing on a flat bench or on a block. On the bench, the plates will go below your feet, and the movement will be several inches longer.

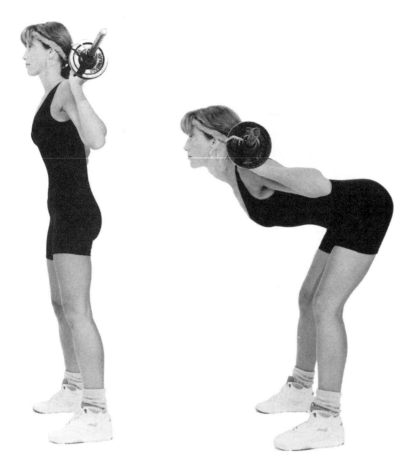

GOOD MORNINGS

Muscles Involved
The erector spinae, with secondary emphasis on the upper back, buttocks, and hamstrings.

Barbell Starting Position
Stand erect with your feet shoulder-width apart and your toes pointed slightly outward. Place a light barbell behind your neck and across your shoulders, steadying it by grasping the bar near the inner plates on each side, palms facing away from your body. Unlock your knees slightly.

Performance
1. Slowly bend forward until your torso is lower than an imaginary line drawn from your hips parallel to the floor. Be sure to keep your back muscles tensed as you descend.
2. Return to the starting point.
3. Repeat as required.

Biomechanical Tips
Unlocking your knees minimizes the possibility of lower-back injury from Good Mornings. As you progress to heavier weights, the bar may begin to cut into your neck rather painfully. Wrapping the bar with a towel will alleviate this problem.

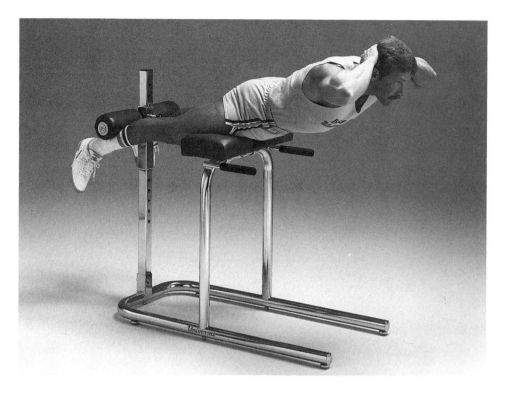

HYPEREXTENSIONS

Muscles Involved
The erector spinae, with secondary emphasis on the upper back, buttocks, and hamstrings.

Starting Position
Get onto the hyperextension bench facedown, your heels hooked securely under the smaller pads and your hips supported by the large pad. Slide forward until the top of your pelvis is directly over the front edge of the large pad. Put your hands behind your neck and interlace your fingers. Finally, sag your body forward until your torso is hanging straight down.

Performance
1. Do a reverse sit-up, arching up backward as high as possible.
2. Return to the initial position.
3. Repeat as required.

Biomechanical Tips
To add resistance on this movement, simply hold a loose barbell plate behind your head as you arch up.

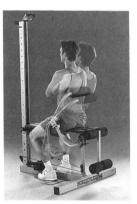

Variation: Nordic® back extension The home unit shown here typifies a seated back-extension movement in which resistance is applied by a pad placed against your back.

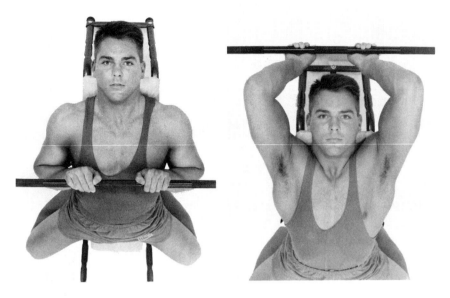

BENT-ARM PULLOVERS

Muscles Involved

The latissimus dorsi, with secondary emphasis on pectorals, forearms, triceps, and deltoids.

Barbell Starting Position

Lie back on a flat bench with your head extending over one end and your feet flat on the floor. Take an overhand grip, your index fingers no more than 6 inches apart, in the middle of a barbell that is resting across the center of your chest. Your palms will be facing forward across the center of your chest and perpendicular to the floor, your elbows pressed against your sides.

Performance

1. Move the bar back in a semicircle from your chest to a point behind and below your head. That will be your full range of motion. Be sure to keep your elbows as close to each other as possible throughout the movement and the bar about an inch from your face as it passes by.

2. Pull the bar back to your chest along the same arc.

3. Repeat the movement as required.

Biomechanical Tips

Never force the barbell any lower behind your head than you are comfortably able to do. Never jerk the weight at this bottom position either, because you could conceivably dislocate your shoulder.

The Cybex® and Nautilus® Pullover machines are excellent alternatives to the free-weight pullover that are often best for the beginner. Just make sure you fit the machine.

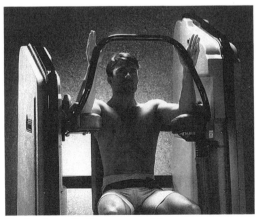

Variation: Pullover machine

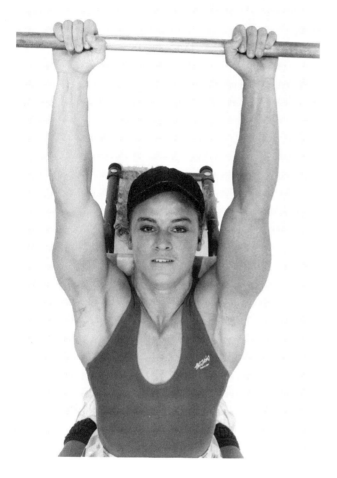

STRAIGHT-ARM PULLOVERS

Muscles Involved
The latissimus dorsi and pectorals, with some emphasis on the trapezius, forearms, and triceps.

Barbell Starting Position
Lie back on a flat bench with your head near one end and your feet flat on the floor. Take an overhand grip in the middle of the barbell handle with your hands 6 inches apart, palms facing forward. Extend your arms until they are straight and the barbell is directly above your chest.

Performance
1. While keeping your elbows locked, allow the barbell to travel in a semicircle back and behind your head as far as you can comfortably go.
2. Return along the same path to the starting position.
3. Repeat as required.

Biomechanical Tips
Each grip width you use on this movement will result in a slightly different stress on the upper back. Try different widths, from hands touching in the middle of the bar to hands that are shoulder-width apart.

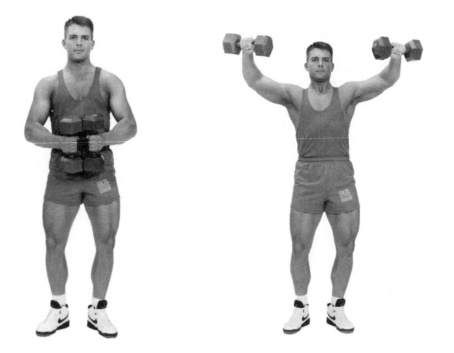

SIDE LATERAL RAISES

Muscles Involved
The medial deltoids, with secondary emphasis on trapezius and anterior deltoids.

Dumbbell Starting Position
Stand erect with your feet shoulder-width apart and your toes pointing a little outward. Grasp a dumbbell in each hand, using an overhand grip, with dumbbells touching each other in front of your hips, elbows bent but locked for the duration of the movement.

Performance
1. Raise your arms straight up until your elbows lock and your upper arms are above an imaginary line drawn from your shoulders that's parallel to the floor.
2. Lower your arms to your sides.
3. Repeat as required.

Biomechanical Tips
You can vary hand positions on the dumbbell side-lateral raises, with palms facing down, forward, or up. As you rotate your palms, stress is gradually moved from the medial deltoid to the anterior deltoid.

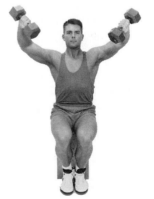

Variation: Seated Side Lateral Raises

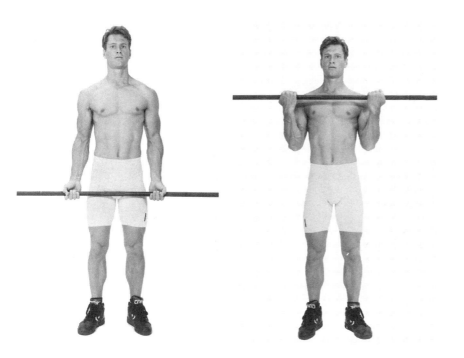

BARBELL BICEPS CURLS

Muscles Involved
The biceps and brachialis, with secondary emphasis on the forearms. Your biceps muscles take part in any sports activity in which your arms must be bent.

Barbell Starting Position
Stand erect with your feet shoulder-width apart and your toes facing slightly outward. Grasp a barbell with an underhand grip, your hands shoulder-width apart and your palms facing away from your ankles. Rest the barbell across the tops of your thighs.

Performance
1. Press your upper arms to your sides and move the bar in a semicircle from the tops of your thighs to your throat, using only the strength of your biceps.
2. Return along the same arc to the starting position.
3. Repeat as required.

Biomechanical Tips
Be careful to keep your upper body rigid and motionless as you do curls. Swinging the torso back and forth removes much of the stress from your biceps.

Home units, such as the one pictured here, offer excellent alternatives to barbell curls.

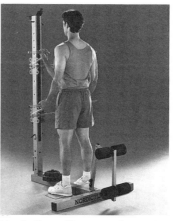

Variation: Home unit- curls

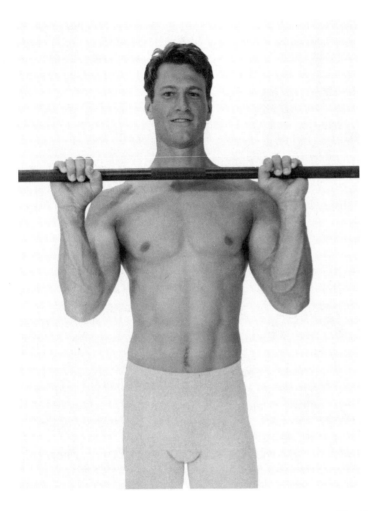

REVERSE BARBELL CURLS

Muscles Involved

The biceps and the brachialis. The wrist extensors play a secondary role in supporting the wrist position. Reverse curls are the most direct exercise you can do for the brachialis muscle, which lies under the biceps on your upper arm.

Barbell Starting Position

Assume exactly the same starting position as you would for a barbell curl, except that your palms should be facing toward your body. This overhand grip is called a reverse grip.

Performance

1. With your upper arms pinned to your sides, move the barbell in a semicircle from the tops of your thighs to your chin.
2. Return along the same arc to the starting point.
3. Repeat as required.

Biomechanical Tips

Many strength trainees have found a grip in the center of the barbell with index fingers about 6 inches apart to be superior to a shoulder-width grip. Try both and decide which you like best.

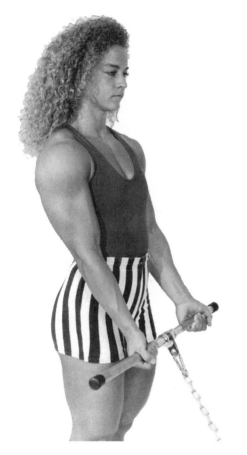

PULLEY CURLS

Muscles Involved

The biceps and the brachialis, with secondary emphasis on the forearm muscles.

Pulley Starting Position

Stand erect with your feet shoulder-width apart and your toes pointed slightly outward, about 6 to 12 inches back from the pulley. Grasp the low pulley handle with an underhand grip, your palms facing away from your body about 12 to 15 inches apart. Rest the handle across your upper thighs in the same position a barbell would be for barbell curls.

Performance

1. Pin your upper arms to your sides and move the pulley handle in a semicircle from your thighs to your chin.
2. Return to start.
3. Repeat the movement as required.

Biomechanical Tips

On this and all other curling movements, be careful to keep your elbows against your sides. Letting them drift outward during a curl will take stress off your biceps, just like it you swing your upper body.

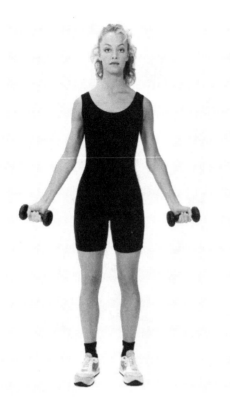 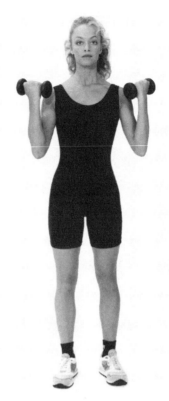

DUMBBELL CURLS

Muscles Involved
The biceps and brachialis, with secondary emphasis on the forearms.

Dumbbell Starting Position
This exercise is done precisely like the barbell curl, except that you use two dumbbells instead of a barbell. Stand erect, a dumbbell in each hand grasped with an underhand grip, your feet shoulder-width apart and your toes pointed slightly outward. Your arms should be hanging straight down at your sides with your palms facing forward.

Performance
1. Keeping your upper arms at your sides, move both dumbbells in a semicircle to your chin, relying solely on biceps power.
2. Lower along the same arc until the dumbbells are back at your sides.
3. Repeat as required.

Biomechanical Tips
Try rotating your hands outward and upward at the top of the curl, which will result in a superior biceps contraction. This is called supination: the biceps supinates as well as flexes the lower arm toward the upper arm. To clarify, the palm of your right hand will be facing straight forward at the beginning of a curl. As the dumbbell goes up, gradually turn your thumb out to the right until your right hand has been twisted as far as possible clockwise. At the same time, your left hand would be twisted in a counterclockwise direction.

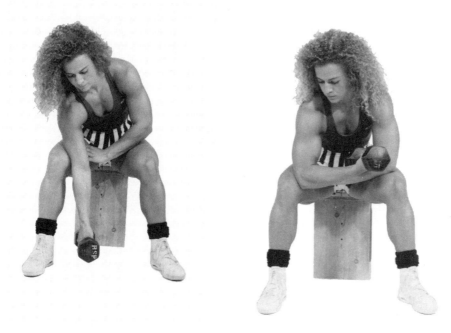

CONCENTRATION CURLS

Muscles Involved
The biceps and brachialis, with secondary emphasis on the forearms.

Dumbbell Starting Position
Sitting, a dumbbell grasped with an underhand grip in your right hand. Your upper arm should be pressed against the inside of your thigh and the dumbbell should hang toward the floor.

Performance
1. With your upper arm remaining against the inside of your thigh, move dumbbell in a semicircle to your chin.
2. Lower along the same arc until the dumbbell is back at the starting position.
3. Repeat as required.
4. Move to the opposite side and repeat the exercise.

Biomechanical Tips
Concentration is the key, using imagery to place stress on your biceps as it draws the dumbbell toward your shoulder.

This is one exercise where machines are particularly effective.

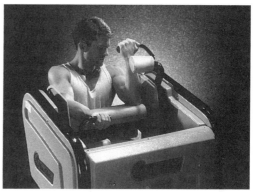

Variation: Nautilus concentration curl The Nautilus® machine offers an advantage of locking the arm in the appropriate position to maximize concentration on the biceps.

TRUNK ROTATION: ISOLATION EXERCISES

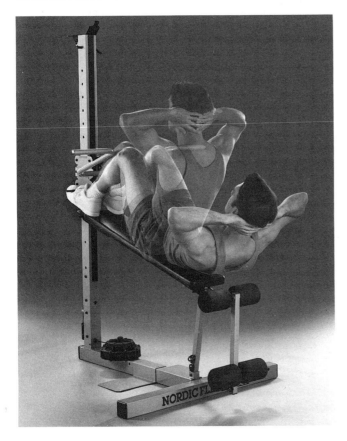

SIT-UPS

Muscles Involved
The frontal abdominals and the hip flexors (psoas and iliacus).

Starting Position
Lie down on your back on a decline sit-up board and hook your feet under the foot straps or rollers. Bend your knees at a 30-degree angle and interlace your fingers behind your head.

Performance
1. Curl your torso up until your elbows touch your knees. By curling up, I mean sequentially lifting your torso up, starting with your upper back, then the middle of your back, and finally your lower back.

2. Return in the opposite sequence (lower back, middle back, upper back) to the starting point.

3. Repeat as required.

Biomechanical Tips
Bending your legs eases strain on your lower back when doing sit-ups. When you are performing sit-ups correctly, your movements will be slow and controlled. Jerking your torso upright (like many ill-informed strength trainees do) is a total waste of movement.

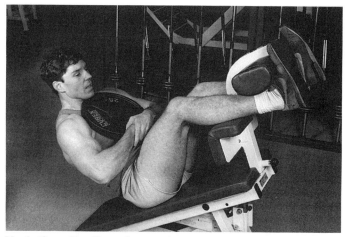

Variation: Decline sit-up with weight As you're
able to perform 8 to 10 reps at a maximum-decline
board, add resistance by holding a barbell plate on

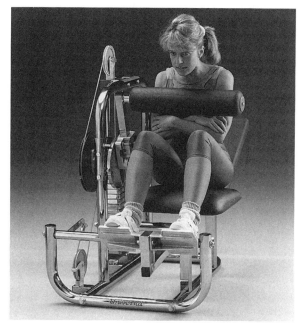

Variation: Universal® Abdominal Machine
A machine such as the Universal® Abdominal
machine pictured here offers an excellent means of
adding resistance to the exercise movement.

PUSH: ISOLATION EXERCISES

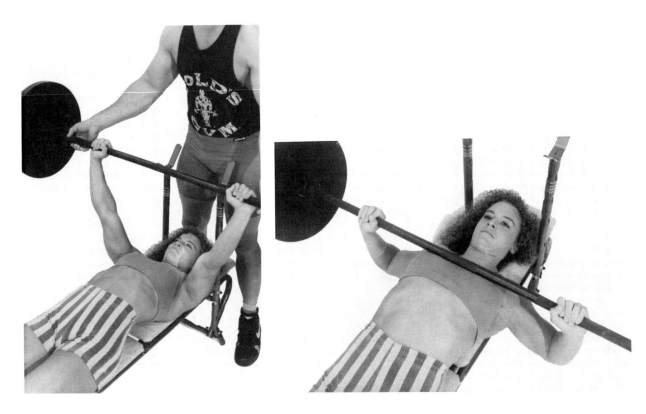

BENCH PRESS

Muscles Involved

The pectorals and deltoids, with significant emphasis on triceps. The forearm muscles and latissimus dorsi act as stabilizing muscles.

Barbell Starting Position

Lie back on a flat bench with your head near one end and your feet flat on the floor. Take a shoulder-width overhand grip on a barbell handle, palms facing forward perpendicular to the floor. Support the barbell at arm's length directly over your chest, keeping your arms straight.

Performance

1. Bend your elbows and let the bar or handles descend to chest level.
2. Press back to the starting position by straightening your arms.
3. Repeat for the required number of sets.

Biomechanical Tips

The movement works the same muscles on both the horizontal (the Universal® Chest Press machine) and the seated machine (Cybex® Chest Press) as illustrated.

**Variation: Universal®
DVR Chest Press.
Starting position:** Lie
back on the flat bench at
the bench-press station,
with your head at one
end of the bench and
your feet flat on the
floor. Take a shoulder-
width overhand grip on
the handles, palms
perpendicular to the
floor. Straighten your
arms so that you are
supporting the handles
at arm's length directly
over your chest.

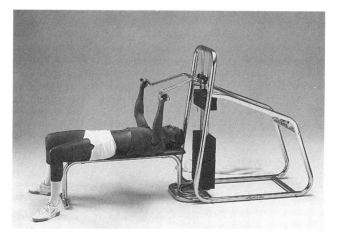

**Variation: Cybex®
Chest Press.
Instructions:** Adjust the
seat height so that
handles are
approximately even with
the sternum. Push the
foot-lever advance
toward the floor to
advance handles to a
comfortable start
position. Select a
neutral or barbell grip.
Slowly release the foot-
lever advance and place
your feet on the foot
platform or the floor.
Start movement by
pressing handles
forward with a smooth,
continuous motion. Do
not lock out elbows at
finish position. Slowly
return to the start
position. When finished,
depress the foot-lever
advance to its start
positions.

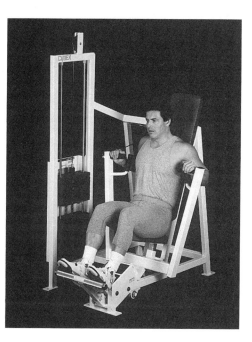

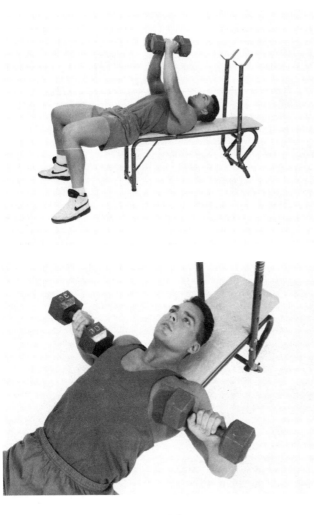

DUMBBELL BENCH PRESS

Muscles Involved

The pectorals and deltoids, with significant emphasis on triceps.

Starting Position

Lie back on flat bench with your head near one end and your feet flat on the floor. Grip a dumbbell in each hand, palms facing forward. Support the dumbbells at arm's length directly over your chest, keeping your arms straight.

Performance

1. Bend your elbows and let the dumbbells descend to chest level, palms facing forward.
2. Press back to the starting position by straightening your arms.
3. Repeat for the required number of sets.

Biomechanical Tips

As you lower the dumbbells from the straight-arm position, the dumbbells make a 90-degree turn so that they are perpendicular to your body as they reach your chest.

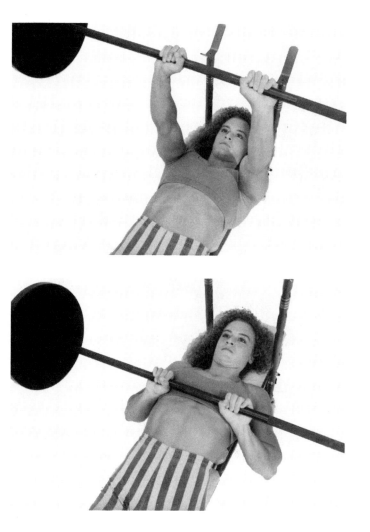

CLOSE GRIP BENCH PRESS

Muscles Involved
The pectorals and deltoids, with significant emphasis on triceps.

Starting Position
Lie back on flat bench with your head near one end and your feet flat on the floor. With an overhand grip in the middle of the barbell handle, hands 6 inches apart and palms facing forward, extend your arms until they are locked out straight over your chest.

Performance
1. Bend your elbows and let the bar or handles descend to chest level.
2. Press back to the starting position by straightening your arms.
3. Repeat for the required number of sets.

Biomechanical Tips
The narrower your grip when bench-pressing, the more stress is shifted to the middle part of your pectorals (the muscle nearer your sternum). With a narrower grip, the triceps also come increasingly into play.

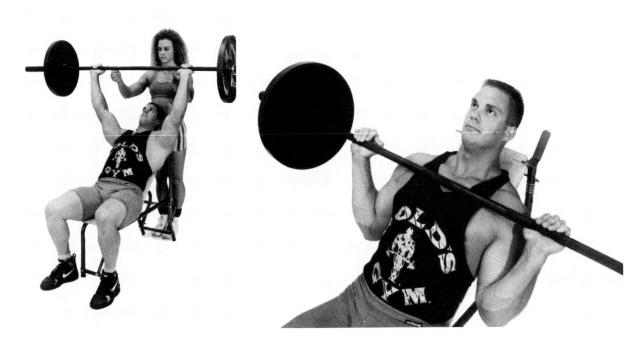

INCLINE BENCH PRESS

Muscles Involved

The upper pectorals, deltoids, and triceps, with secondary emphasis on the lower pectorals.

Barbell Starting Position

Lie back on a 45-degree incline bench, with your feet flat on the pedals or floor. Take a shoulder-width overhand grip on the barbell, palms facing your body and the barbell lying across your thighs. Bring the weight to the base of your neck so that your elbows are directly below the barbell handle.

Performance

1. Push the weight straight up from the chest until your elbows lock.
2. Lower to the starting point.
3. Repeat as required.

Biomechanical Tips

The elbows must be kept directly under the weight at all times because this position puts maximum stress on the pectorals and deltoids. While flat bench presses were once the favorite chest exercise of football players, inclines are now most popular because they more closely simulate the angle at which the arms are extended in driving into an opponent.

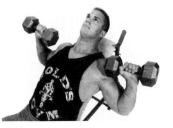

Variation: Incline-bench dumbbell press Incline-bench dumbbell press. This variation uses dumbbells instead of the barbell. Except for the incline, follow the instructions for the dumbbell bench press on page 160.

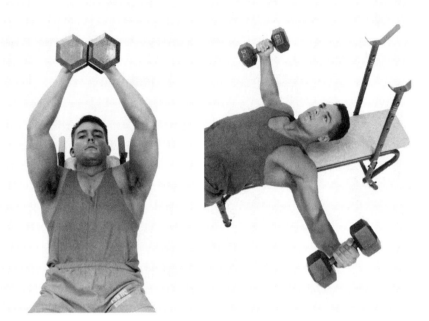

CHEST FLY ON FLAT OR INCLINE BENCH

Muscles Involved
The pectorals when done on a flat bench, with secondary emphasis on deltoids. On an incline bench you can isolate the movement more to your upper pectorals, while on a decline bench the emphasis shifts to your lower pectorals.

Dumbbell Starting Position
Lie back on a flat or incline bench with your head at one end and feet flat on the floor. Grasp two dumbbells with a parallel grip. Hold them at arm's length straight over your chest, the handles parallel and the inner edges touching each other. Your palms should face inward. Your elbows will remain locked but slightly bent throughout the movement.

Performance
1. Move the dumbbells out to the sides in semicircles to as low a point as possible.
2. Return to the starting position through the same semicircular path.
3. Repeat as required.

Variations
Two popular machine equivalents, Cybex® and Universal®, are pictured below. Consult the machine-version manuals for correct procedures.

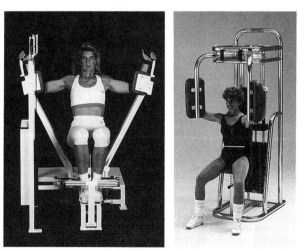

Cybex® Chest Fly Machine
Universal® DVR Vertical Chest Bench

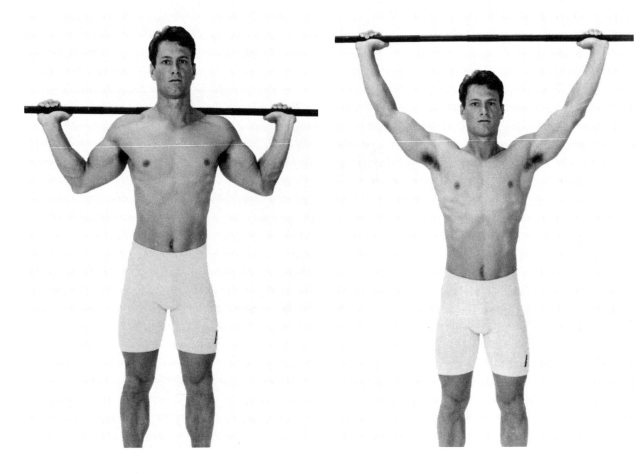

PRESS BEHIND NECK

Muscles Involved
The frontal deltoids, with secondary emphasis on the rest of the deltoids, triceps, and trapezius.

Barbell Starting Position
Stand erect with your feet a shoulder-width apart and your toes angled slightly outward. Place a barbell behind your neck and across your shoulders. Grasp it with an overhand grip, hands about 6 inches wider than your shoulders on each side, palms facing forward.

Performance
1. Push the barbell straight up until your elbows lock and the weight is directly above your head.
2. Bend your elbows and return the weight to the starting point.
3. Repeat as required.

Biomechanical Tips
To make this a better exercise, sit on a bench or chair so that you don't use your legs to help you lift. You'll find that you use less weight this way.

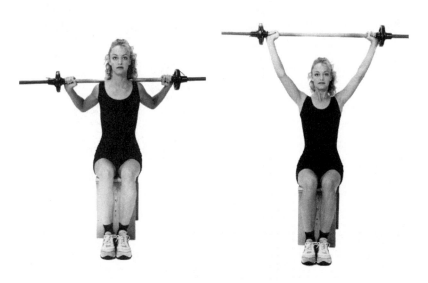

Variation: Seated press behind neck Follow the same instructions for this exercise as you did for the standing version.

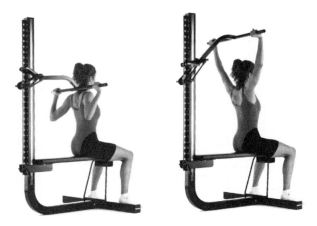

Soloflex® Home Unit You can also do this exercise without a spotter, on the Soloflex® machine as shown in the illustrations.

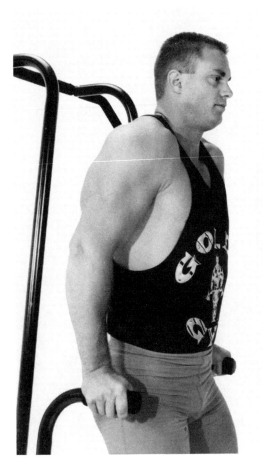

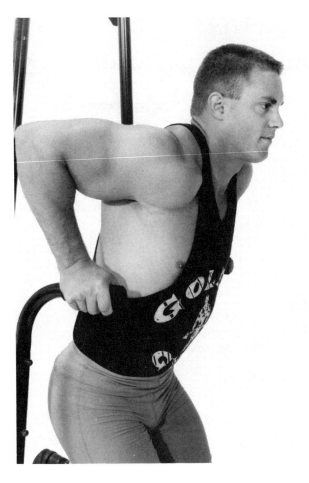

DIPS

Muscles Involved
The lower pectorals, deltoids, and triceps, with secondary emphasis on upper pectorals and latissimus dorsi.

Starting Position
Grip the ends of a set of parallel bars with a parallel grip, your palms facing each other. Support your full body weight on your hands, with your arms straight along the sides of your body. If you have to, bend your knees to avoid touching your feet on the floor.

Performance
1. Bend your arms and lower your shoulders to the bars.
2. Descend as low as you can without losing control and then press back up to the starting point.
3. Repeat as required.

Biomechanical Tips
For proper muscle action in this movement, it is vital to keep your elbows centered above the bars at all times. For extra pectoral stress, lean forward with your upper body and flex about 10 degrees at your waist. For more triceps emphasis, do the movement with your upper body as upright as possible.

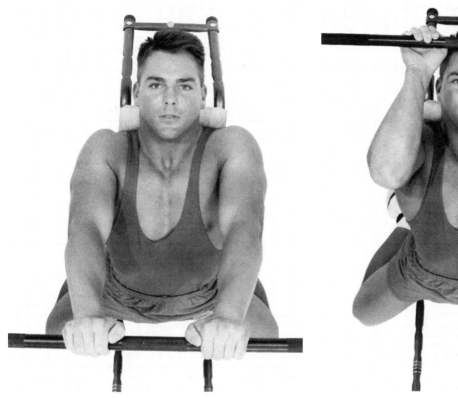
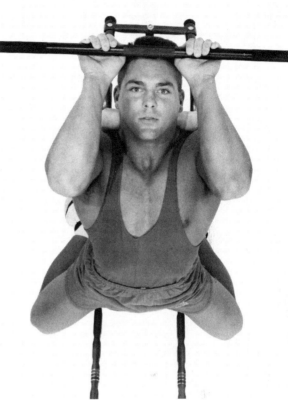

LYING BARBELL TRICEPS EXTENSIONS

Muscles Involved
The triceps on the backs of your upper arms, with secondary emphasis on forearms.

Barbell Starting Position
Lie back on a flat bench with your feet flat on the floor on either side of the bench to balance your body. Take a narrow overhand grip (6 inches or less between your hands) on a barbell, being careful to balance your grip in the middle of the bar. Start with the barbell grasped with arms straight over your chest, palms perpendicular to the floor, and facing toward your feet.

Performance
1. Keeping your upper arms absolutely stationary, lower the barbell in a semicircle from the starting point until it touches your forehead.
2. Return along the same arc with triceps strength until you are again back to the starting position.
3. Repeat as required.

Biomechanical Tips
Never allow your elbows to flare out to the sides as you do triceps extensions because this movement will take considerable stress off your triceps.

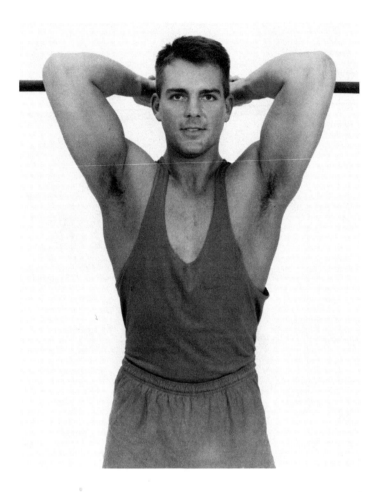

STANDING TRICEPS EXTENSIONS

Muscles Involved
The triceps, with secondary emphasis on the forearms.

Barbell Starting Position
Take a narrow overhand grip on a barbell. Your hands should be no more than 6 inches apart, and your palms should be facing forward. Stand erect with your feet at shoulder width, toes pointed slightly outward, and swing the barbell up until your arms are extended straight overhead.

Performance
1. Lock your upper arms against the sides of your head. With your upper arms motionless, lower the bar in a semicircle by bending your elbows until the bar touches the back of your neck.
2. Return to the starting position.
3. Repeat as required.

Biomechanical Tips
Remember that your elbows shouldn't flare out and away from your head, and your upper arms must remain motionless.

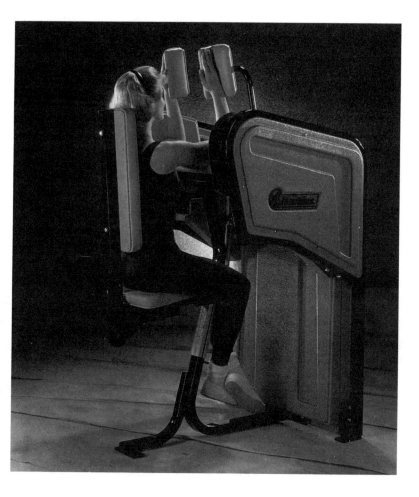

NAUTILUS® TRICEPS EXTENSIONS

Muscles Involved
The triceps, with secondary emphasis on the forearms. Triceps strength is essential in any athletic activity in which you straighten your arm from a bent position, such as throwing a ball or javelin.

Starting Position
Adjust the seat up or down on the Nautilus Multi-Triceps machine so that the backs of your upper arms rest comfortably on the large lower pad.

Performance
1. Straighten your arms with triceps power.
2. Return to the starting position.
3. Repeat as required.
4. Let the weights return over your head before you get off the machine.

Biomechanical Tips
Be sure to keep your elbows anchored to the elbow pads throughout the exercise. You can also occasionally try this movement with your palms facing away to attack the triceps from a slightly different angle.

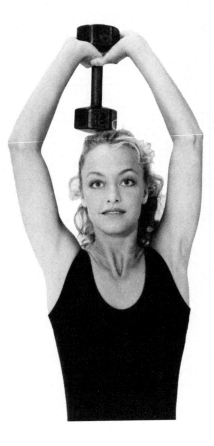

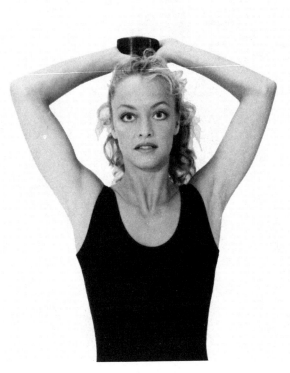

DUMBBELL TRICEPS EXTENSIONS

Muscles Involved

The triceps, with secondary emphasis on the fore-arms.

Starting Position

Stand with your feet about shoulder-width apart. Grasp a single dumbbell in both hands, with your fingers interlaced, and extend your arms directly overhead until your elbows are locked. The dumbbell handle should be perpendicular to the floor, with your hands touching the underside of the top plate, and the bottom plate hanging down below your hands.

Performance

1. Keep your upper arms stationary and bend at the elbows to let the dumbbell move in a semi-circle from the starting point until it touches the back of your neck.

2. Extend your arms back to the start with triceps power, being careful not to move your upper arms.

3. Repeat as required.

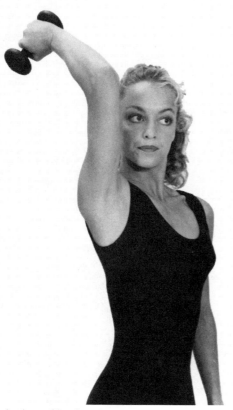

Variation: Single-arm dumbbell triceps extensions For variety you can also do dumbbell triceps extensions with one arm at a time or you can do the exercise with two dumbells at once, one in each hand.

SPECIALTY EXERCISES

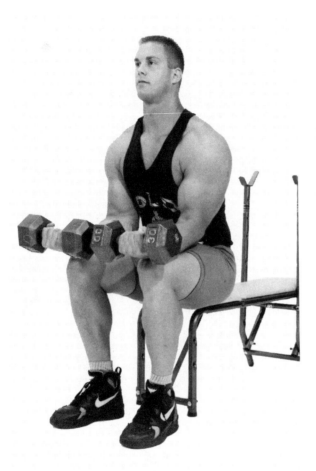 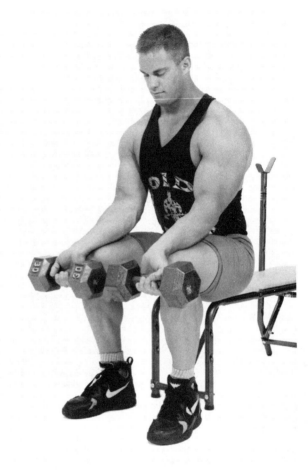

DUMBBELL WRIST CURLS

Muscles Involved
All of the muscles of your forearms.

Dumbbell Starting Position
Sit upright at the end of a flat bench and grasp a pair of dumbbells in your hands, palms up and forearms resting on your thighs. Your wrists should extend past your knees.

Performance
1. Sag both wrists down toward the floor as far as possible, keeping your forearms stationary.
2. Curl both wrists up as high as possible.
3. Lower.
4. Repeat as required.

Biomechanical Tips
For better concentration, do one arm at a time.

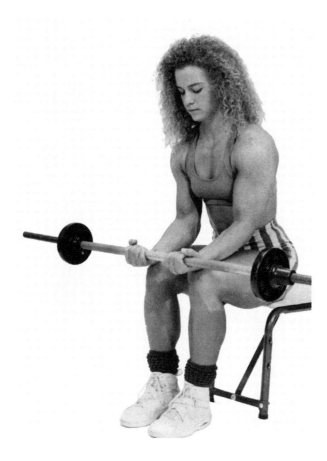

BARBELL WRIST CURLS

Muscles Involved
All of the muscles of your forearms.

Barbell Starting Position
Sit on the end of a flat bench, your forearms resting on your thighs. Grasp a barbell in your hands with your palms up. Use a shoulder-width grip and let your wrists extend beyond your knees.

Performance
1. Sag your wrists down toward the floor as far as they will go and then curl the weight up as high as you can.
2. Lower.
3. Repeat as required. Be sure you move nothing but your wrists on this exercise.

Biomechanical Tips
When you have done 2 or 3 sets of wrist curls with your palms facing up, turn your palms down and do a few more sets. You will find that you can use about half as much weight with palms down as you used with them up. Wrist curls with palms up work the insides of your forearms; those with palms down, the outsides of your forearms.

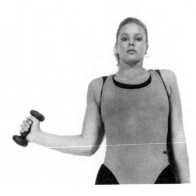

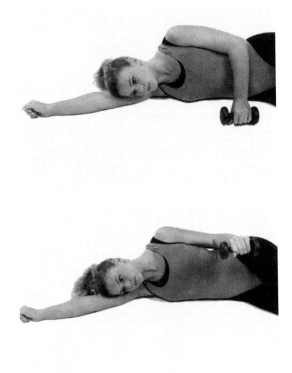

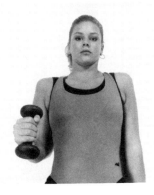

ROTATOR CUFF SERIES

Training Tip

This set of exercises is particularly valuable to any athlete who relies on overhand throws in his athletic event—especially quarterbacks, pitchers, and javelin throwers. The exercises strengthen the muscles that stabilize the shoulder, helping to prevent career-threatening rotator cuff injuries.

Exercise One

1. Lie on your back on the floor, elbow at your side, hand gripping a dumbbell positioned as shown below.

2. Lift the dumbbell through an arc until your hand is directly above your elbow. Keep your upper arm and elbow on the floor throughout the lift.

3. Lower the dumbbell to the floor through the same arc. That's a rep.

Exercise Two

1. Lie on your side on the floor, elbow pressed against your side, hand gripping a dumbbell positioned on the floor as shown.

2. Lift the dumbbell through an arc until your forearm is parallel to the floor. Keep your upper arm and elbow pressed against the side of your body throughout the lift.

3. Lower the dumbbell to the floor through the same arc. That's a rep.

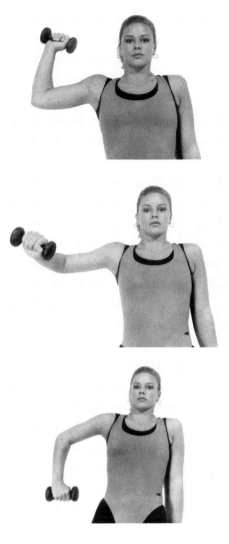

Exercise Three

1. Lie on your back on the floor, upper arm at a 90-degree angle to your body. Grip a dumbbell positioned above your head as shown.

2. Keeping your elbow at a right angle and your arm pressed against the floor, move the dumbbell through a 180-degree arc until the dumbbell touches the floor next to your hip.

3. Return the dumbbell through the same arc to the starting position. That's a rep.

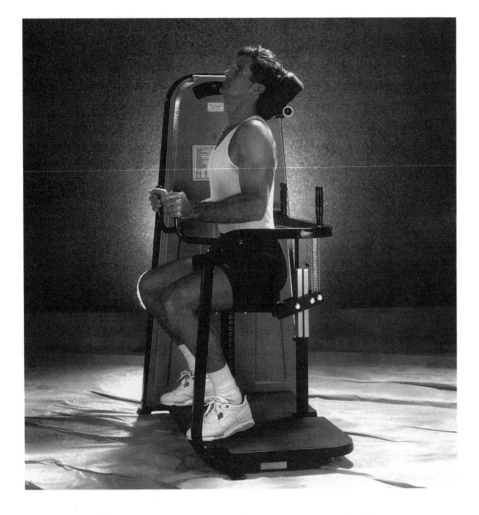

NAUTILUS® 4-WAY NECK MACHINE

Muscles Involved

All of the muscles of the neck (flexors, extensors, and lateral flexors), with secondary emphasis on the trapezius.

Starting Position

Sit facing the machine, with the seat adjusted at a height that allows you to place the front of your head directly on the pads. Lean into the pads and let your head come forward to your chest.

Performance

1. Use your neck to move the head forward as far as possible.
2. Allow your head to return to the initial position.
3. Repeat the movement with the pads behind and on alternate sides of your head.

Biomechanical Tips

These neck exercises are particularly important for athletes in contact sports where the head and neck are involved.

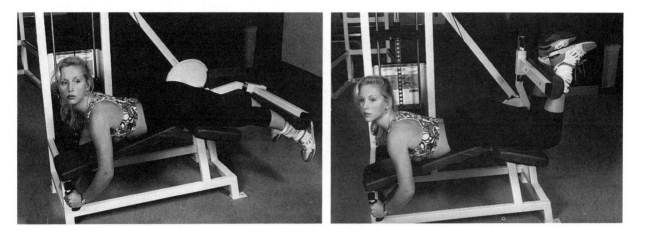

CYBEX® LEG CURL

Muscles Involved
The hamstrings, with secondary emphasis on the calves and buttocks. Hamstrings strength is helpful in all athletic movements where you bend your legs from a straight position, such as sprinting and jumping.

Cybex Starting Position
Lie facedown or chestdown on a leg-curl machine with your knees off the bench. Adjust the leg pad so that it is positioned just above the Achilles tendon. Grasp the handles under the bench to steady your body.

Performance
1. Bend your legs at the knees as much as possible, using hamstring strength. Curl the heels to buttocks with a smooth, controlled motion.
2. Lower to the starting position.
3. Repeat as required.

Biomechanical Tips
It is also important not to lift your hips up from the bench as you do leg curls because this will shorten your range of motion.

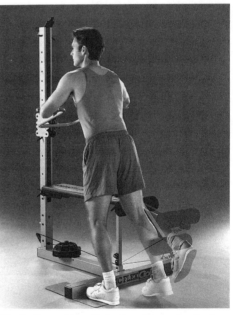

Variation: Nordic® standing single-leg curl A standing leg curl allows for greater concentration by limiting the movement to one leg at a time. The exercise is available with the Nordic® and with many other commercial units. All are similar in concept.

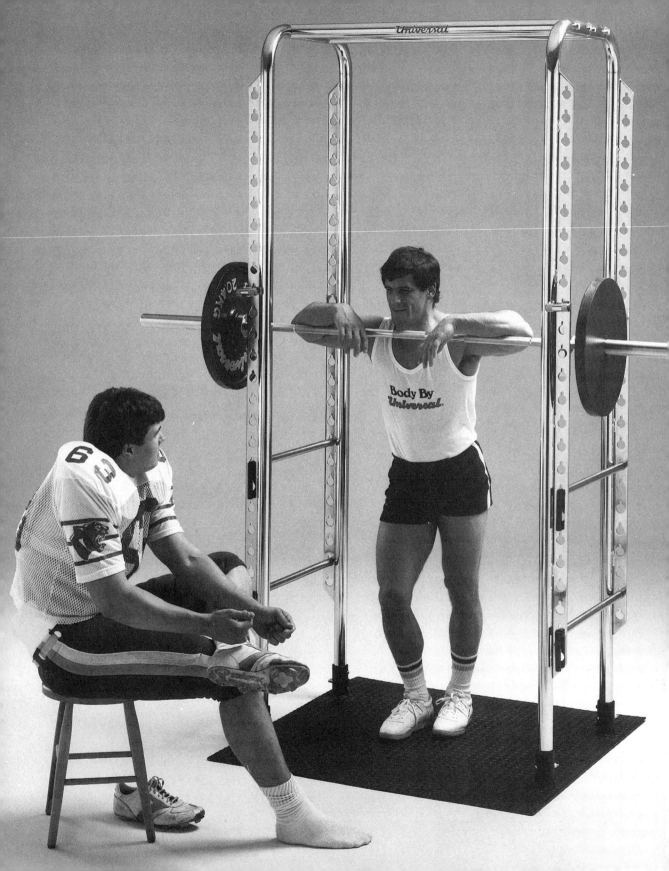

10
Packaged Sports Programs

In this chapter you're going to be able to choose from thirty sport-specific strength programs, each tailored to an individual sport, and, in some instances, to specific activities within general sports categories. I call them Packaged Programs.

All programs are equally suited for male and female athletes and can be used throughout the year. Or refer to chapter 5, under "Seasonal Alterations," to adjust the program to coincide with the off-season or competitive-season demands of your sport. And if you're new to strength training or coming back from a layoff, reread chapter 7 to refresh your understanding of the Basic Movement Program, the core of all Packaged Programs.

If you wish, these programs can be a foundation for an individualized training program, enhanced with the suggestions provided in chapters 8 and 9. An individually designed schedule will produce superior results.

WHAT'S IN A PACKAGED PROGRAM?

Each Packaged Program has the following two elements:

1. The Basic Movement Program and
2. Additional exercises, selected to have the greatest impact on the sport in question.

WHERE TO BEGIN

If you have already established your Basic Movement Program, simply add the additional exercises listed for your sport to your Program Chart (chapter 7, page 127).

If you're new to strength training, return to chapter 7 and establish a Basic Movement Program before tackling the Packaged Programs. Jumping into the Packaged Program without prior training experience is likely to be too intense and confusing. Start out right, make the first several months a positive experience, and you will likely stick to strength training for years to come.

· Modifying the Package

Chapter 8 outlines means of modifying exercises and programs to meet your individual athletic needs. It's okay to modify the Package according to the suggested guidelines. In fact, rereading that chapter at this point—it's a short chapter—will help you understand the reasoning for the exercise selection contained in your Packaged Program.

Here are the Packaged Programs:

THE PROGRAMS

Archery

Primary Strength Needs:
Pull, leg strength, triceps and shoulder strength, torso stabilization, string grip and release.

Page Exercise	Sets	Reps
87 Basic Movement Program	5	6
143 Bent Row with Dumbbell	3	6–10
145 Stiff-Legged Deadlift	3	6–10
172 Wrist Curl	3	6–10

Baseball and Softball

General Strength Needs:
Leg and hip thrust, upper-body pull and thrust, torso rotation, torso stabilization, and knee lift.

Page Exercise	Sets	Reps
87 Basic Movement Program	5	6
145 Stiff-Legged Deadlift	3	6–10
158 Bench Press	3	6–10
148 Bent-Arm Pullover	3	6–10

Primary Strength Needs for Batting:

Forearm, wrist, and hand strength.

Page Exercise	Sets	Reps
87 Basic Movement Program	5	6
172 Wrist Curl	3	6–10
148 Bent-Arm Pullover	3	6–10

Primary Strength Needs for Pitching:

Forearm-wrist action, hand strength, shoulder girdle.

Page Exercise	Sets	Reps
87 Basic Movement Program	5	6
92 *Leg Drive Movement	5	6
170 Dumbbell Triceps Extensions	3	6–10
172 Wrist Curls	3	6–10
174 Rotator Cuff Series	3	6–10

Primary Strength Needs for Throwing:

Shoulder, triceps, legs.

Page Exercise	Sets	Reps
87 Basic Movement Program	5	6
174 Rotator Cuff Series	3	6–10
148 Bent-Arm Pullover	3	6–10
167–171 Triceps Extensions	3	6–10

Basketball

I was one of the first basketball players to go on a weight program. Coaches always told us not to touch weights, that weight would ruin our shooting touch. I was 24 years old and had won the rebounding title, but I also was 215 pounds. I wanted to be the pounder, not take a pounding every night. I worked with a guy named Alvin Roy, who was a strength coach at LSU. My coach and owner didn't like it, especially when I showed up at 240 pounds. But I felt my hands, my arms, everything was stronger. With today's conditioning programs, I'd play at 265.

Bob Petit, *Tall Tales,* by Terry Pluto

Primary Strength Needs:

Leg and hip thrust, knee strength, upper-body thrust and pull, back strength, hand strength, and ankle strength.

Page Exercise	Sets	Reps
87 Basic Movement Program	5	6
92 *Leg Drive Movement	5	6
133 Partial Squat	3	6–10
161 Close-Grip Bench Press	3	6–10
140 Lat-Machine Pulldown	3	6–10
145 Stiff-Legged Deadlift	3	6–10
134–135 Calf Raise	3	6–10

Bowling

Primary Strength Needs:

Hip and leg thrust, upper-body pull and thrust, torso stabilization, torso extension, forearm and wrist strength, and elbow and arm strength.

Page Exercise	Sets	Reps
87 Basic Movement Program	5	6
143 Bent-over Dumbbell Row	3	6–10
144 Upright Row	3	6–10
145 Stiff-Legged Deadlift	3	6–10
172 Wrist Curl	3	6–10
154–155 Dumbbell Biceps Curl	3	6–10

*Include an additional movement exercise from this Basic Movement group.

Boxing

Primary Strength Needs:
Hip and leg thrust, upper-body thrust (punch), torso rotation, upper-body pull, wrist extension, and back stabilization.

Page Exercise	Sets	Reps
87 Basic Movement Program	5	6
92 *Leg Drive	5	6
158 *Push	5	6
160 Dumbbell Bench Press	3	6–10
156–157 Sit-up	3	6–10
172 Wrist Curl	3	6–10
143 Bent-over Dumbbell Row	3	6–10
145 Stiff-Legged Deadlift	3	6–10
148 Bent-Arm Pullover	3	6–10

Climbing

Primary Strength Needs:
Hip and leg drive, upper-body pull, shoulder and wrist strength.

Page Exercise	Sets	Reps
87 Basic Movement Program	5	6
99 *Pull	5	6
166 Dips	3	6–10
177 Leg Curl	3	6–10
150 Side Lateral Raises	3	6–10

Cycling

Primary Strength Needs:
Hip and leg drive, upper-body pull, knee strength, torso stabilization, rotational strength, and triceps and shoulder strength.

Page Exercise	Sets	Reps
87 Basic Movement Program	5	6
92 *Leg Drive	5	6
145 Stiff-Legged Deadlift	3	6–10
166 Dip	3	6–10
177 Leg Curl	3	6–10

Diving

Primary Strength Needs:
Leg strength and torso stabilization.

Page Exercise	Sets	Reps
87 Basic Movement Program	5	6
145 Stiff-Legged Deadlift	3	6–10
136 Leg Extensions	3	6–10
150 Side Lateral Raises	3	6–10

Fencing

Primary Strength Needs:
Hip and leg thrust, knee strength, torso stabilization, upper-body thrust and pull, hand strength, and wrist strength.

Page Exercise	Sets	Reps
87 Basic Movement Program	5	6
92 *Leg Drive (Lunge)	5	6
161 Close Grip Bench Press	3	6–10
145 Stiff-Legged Deadlift	3	6–10
144 Upright Row	3	6–10
172 Wrist Curl	3	6–10

*Include an additional movement exercise from this Basic Movement group.

Football

General Strength Needs for Linemen:
Hip and leg thrust, upper-body pull and thrust, back strength–extension, and torso rotational strength.

Page	Exercise	Sets	Reps
87	Basic Movement Program	5	6
92	*Leg Drive (Leg Press)	5	6
148	Bent-Arm Pullover	3	6–10
145	Stiff-Legged Deadlift	3	6–10
176	Neck Machine	3	6–10
158	Bench Press	3	6–10

Primary Strength Needs for Kickers and Punters:
Leg thrust and knee strength.

Page	Exercise	Sets	Reps
87	Basic Movement Program	5	6
92	*Leg Drive	5	6
106	Knee Lift with Cable	5	6
136	Leg Extension	3	6–10
177	Leg Curl	3	6–10

Primary Strength Needs for Centers:
Upper-body pull and thrust, elbow support, and wrist, hand, and finger strength.

Page	Exercise	Sets	Reps
87	Basic Movement Program	5	6
92	*Leg Drive	5	6
148	Bent-Arm Pullover	3	6–10
167	Barbell Triceps Extension	3	6–10
172	Wrist Curl	3	6–10

Primary Strength Needs for Quarterbacks:
Upper-body throwing strength, shoulder development, wrist and hand strength, elbow support, leg thrust, and knee strength.

To acquire this balance of body strength, do the basic strength-training module plus the following movement exercises:

Page	Exercise	Sets	Rep
87	Basic Movement Program	5	6
167–171	Tricep Extensions	3	6–10
172	Wrist Curl	3	6–10
174	Rotator Cuff Series	3	6–10
177	Leg Curl	3	6–10
148	Bent-Arm Pullover	3	6–10

Primary Strength Needs for Running Backs, Defensive Backs, and Linebackers:
Hip and leg thrust, torso rotational strength, and knee strength.

Page	Exercise	Sets	Reps
87	Basic Movement Program	5	6
92	*Leg Drive	5	6
177	Leg Curl	3	6–10
145	Stiff-Legged Deadlift	3	6–10
158	Bench Press	3	6–10

*Include an additional movement exercise from this Basic Movement group.

Golf

Primary Strength Needs:
Hips and leg thrust, torso rotation and stabilization, shoulder strength, back extension, wrist and forearm strength, hand strength, and upper-body pull.

Page Exercise	Sets	Reps
87 Basic Movement Program	5	6
150 Side Lateral Raises	5	6–10
144 Upright Row	3	6–10
145 Stiff-Legged Deadlift	3	6–10
172 Wrist Curl	3	6–10

Gymnastics

Consult with your coach to identify the muscles that are important to your specialty. You and your coach can determine which muscle groups are weak, then choose one or two exercises to do for each group.

Hockey

Primary Strength Needs:
Arm strength, leg power, and wrist strength.

Page Exercise	Sets	Reps
87 Basic Movement Program	5	6
92 *Leg Drive	5	6
150 Side Lateral Raises	3	6–10
177 Leg Curls	3	6–10
172 Wrist Curls	3	6–10

Martial Arts

Primary Strength Needs:
Torso rotation, hip and leg thrust, upper-body pull and thrust, and back strength–extension.

Page Exercise	Sets	Reps
87 Basic Movement Program	5	6
92 *Leg Drive	5	6
99 *Pull	5	6
145 Stiff-Legged Deadlift	3	6–10
148 Bent-Arm Pullover	3	6–10
136 Leg Extensions	3	6–10

Racquetball and Squash

Primary Strength Needs:
Hip and leg thrust, torso rotation, torso stabilization, knee strength, forearm and wrist strength, back strength–extension, upper-body thrust and pull, and hand strength.

Page Exercise	Sets	Reps
87 Basic Movement Program	5	6
177 Leg Curl	3	6–10
143 Bent-Over Dumbbell Row	3	6–10
145 Stiff-Legged Deadlift	3	6–10
172 Wrist Curl	3	6–10
174 Rotator Cuff	3	6–10

*Include an additional movement exercise from this Basic Movement group.

Rowing and Kayaking

Primary Strength Needs:
Hip and leg thrust, upper-body pull and thrust, back strength—extension, and torso stabilization.

Page Exercise	Sets	Reps
87 Basic Movement Program	5	6
102 *Pull (seated cable long pull)	5	6
145 Stiff-Legged Deadlift	3	6–10
148 Bent-Arm Pullover	3	6–10
143 Bent-Over Dumbbell Row	3	6–10

Skating

Primary Strength Needs:
Hip and leg thrust, back strength—extension, forearm strength, knee strength.

Page Exercise	Sets	Reps
87 Basic Movement Program	5	6–10
92 *Leg Drive	5	6
156–157 Sit-ups	3	6–10
134–135 Calf Raises	3	6–10
177 Leg Curl	5	6–10
147 Hyperextensions	3	6–10

Nordic Skiing

Primary Strength Needs:
Hip and leg thrust, upper-body pull and thrust, back strength—extension, forearm strength, knee strength.

Page Exercise	Sets	Reps
87 Basic Movement Program	5	6–10
92 *Leg Drive	5	6
161 Close Grip Bench Press	3	6–10
143 Bent-Over Dumbbell Row	3	6–10
177 Leg Curl	5	6–10
172 Wrist Curl	3	6–10

Soccer

Primary Strength Needs:
Leg and hip thrust, upper-body pull and thrust, hamstring strength, back strength—extension, torso rotational strength, torso stabilization, and knee strength.

Page Exercise	Sets	Reps
87 Basic Movement Program	5	6
92 *Leg Drive	5	6
177 Leg Curl	3	6–10
145 Stiff-Legged Deadlift	3	6–10
134–135 Calf Raises	3	6–10

Swimming

Primary Strength Needs:
Hip and leg thrust, knee strength—flexion, torso stabilization, pectoral development, upper-body pull, and shoulder-girdle strength.

Page Exercise	Sets	Reps
87 Basic Movement Program	5	6
39 Swim Trainer	3	6–10
163 Chest Fly	3	6–10
147 Hyperextensions	3	6–10
174 Rotator Cuff series	3	6–10

*Include an additional movement exercise from this Basic Movement group.

Tennis

Primary Strength Needs:

Hip and leg thrust, knee strength, torso rotational strength, torso stabilization, upper-body thrust and pull, and forearm and wrist strength.

Page	Exercise	Sets	Reps
87	Basic Movement Program	5	6
92	*Leg Drive	5	6
147	Hyperextensions	3	6–10
143	Bent-Over Dumbbell Row	3	6–10
172	Wrist Curl	3	6–10
144	Upright Row	3	6–10
150	Side Lateral Raises	3	6–10

Track and Field

THROWS—SHOT PUT
DISCUS
JAVELIN

Primary Strength Needs for Throwing:

Leg and hip thrust, torso rotation, upper-body power, back strength–extension, and hand and forearm strength.

Page	Exercise	Sets	Reps
87	Basic Movement Program	5	6
148	Bent-Arm Pullover	3	6–10
145	Stiff-Legged Deadlift	3	6–10
177	Leg Curl	3	6–10
170	Dumbbell Triceps Extensions	3	6–10
172	Wrist Curl	3	6–10

JUMPS

Primary Strength Needs:

Leg and hip strength; torso stabilization and strength.

Page	Exercise	Sets	Reps
87	Basic Movement Program	5	6
92	*Leg Drive	5	6
133	Partial Squat	3	6–10
145	Stiff-Legged Deadlift	3	6–10
134–135	Calf Raises	3	6–10
177	Leg Curl	3	6–10

VAULTERS

Primary Strength Needs:

Leg and hip thrust, hamstring strength, back strength–extension, upper-body pull and thrust, torso rotational strength, and forearm and wrist strength.

Page	Exercise	Sets	Reps
87	Basic Movement Program	5	6
102	*Pull (Seated Cable Long Pull)	5	6
177	Leg Curl	5	6–10
161	Close Grip Bench Press	3	6–10
102	Seated Cable Long Pull	3	6–10
147	Hyperextensions	3	6–10
172	Wrist Curl	3	6–10

*Include an additional movement exercise from this Basic Movement group.

SPRINTS AND HURDLES

Primary Strength Needs:
Leg and hip thrust, calf strength.

Page Exercise	Sets	Reps
87 Basic Movement Program	5	6
92 *Leg Drive	5	6
136 Leg Extensions	3	6–10
177 Leg Curl	3	6–10
134–135 Calf Raises	3	6–10
166 Dip	3	6–10

DISTANCE RUNNING

Primary Strength Needs:
Hip and leg thrust, hamstring and knee strength, ankle and calf strength, and torso stabilization.

Page Exercise	Sets	Reps
87 Basic Movement Program	5	6
177 Leg Curl	3	6–10
145 Stiff-Legged Deadlift	3	6–10
134–135 Calf Raises	3	6–10

TRIATHLON

Primary Strength Needs:
Leg and hip thrust, torso rotational strength and torso stabilization, back strength—extension, and shoulder development.

Page Exercise	Sets	Reps
87 Basic Movement Program	5	6–10
145 Stiff-Legged Deadlift	3	6–10
144 Upright Row	3	6–10
391 Swim Trainer		

Triathletes can refer to the three specific Swimming, Track, and Cycling Programs for additional strength-straining exercises.

Volleyball

Primary Strength Needs:
Hip and leg thrust, upper-body pull and thrust, ankle strength, knee strength, back strength—extension, torso stabilization, and hand and wrist strength.

Page Exercise	Sets	Reps
87 Basic Movement Program	5	6
92 *Leg Drive	5	6
140 Lat Pull-down	3	6–10
148 Bent-Arm Pullover	3	6–10
134–135 Calf Raises	3	6–10
145 Stiff-Legged Deadlift	3	6–10
172 Wrist Curls	3	6–10
147 Hyperextensions	3	6–10

*Include an additional movement exercise from this Basic Movement group.

Water Polo

Primary Strength Needs:
Upper-body strength.

Page Exercise	Sets	Reps
87 Basic Movement Program	5	6
148 Bent-Arm Pullovers	3	6–10
167–171 Triceps Extensions	3	6–10

Water Skiing

Primary Strength Needs:
Upper-body strength, leg and wrist strength.

Page Exercise	Sets	Reps
87 Basic Movement Program	5	6
99 *Pull	5	6
92 *Leg Drive	5	6
172 Wrist Curl	3	6–10

Wrestling

Primary Strength Needs:
Upper-body strength, hip and leg thrust, torso rotational strength, and back strength.

Page Exercise	Sets	Reps
87 Basic Movement Program	5	6
99 *Pull	5	6
92 *Leg Drive	5	6

*Include an additional movement exercise from this Basic Movement group.

Appendix: Exercise Equipment Directory

· **Cybex**®

Lumex Inc.
2100 Smithtown Avenue
P.O. Box 9003
Ronkonkoma, NY 11779-0903

· **Soloflex**®**, Inc.**

Hawthorn Farm Industrial Park
Hillsboro, OR 97124-6494

· **Nautilus**®

Nautilus Acquisition Corporation
709 Powerhouse Road
Independence, VA 24348

· **Nordic Track**®

104 Peavy Road
Chaska, MN 55318

· **Speed City Inc.**

P.O. Box 1059
Portland, OR 97207

· **StairMaster**®

Sports/Medical Products, Inc.
12421 Willows Road NE, Suite 100
Kirkland, WA 98034

· **Universal**® **Gym Equipment, Inc.**

930 27th Avenue S.W.
Box 1270
Cedar Rapids, Iowa 52406

· **Vasa Swim Trainer**

372 Governor Chittenden Road
Williston, Vermont 95495

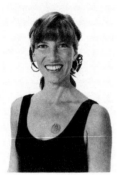

Molly Beauchamp

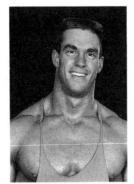

Bruce Budzig

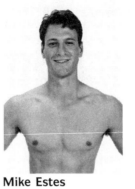

Mike Estes

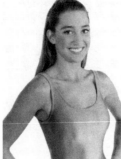

Aubree Knecht

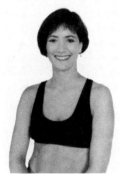

Sheila Kryl

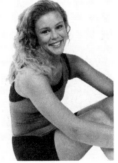

Robin Mitzel

Matt Powers

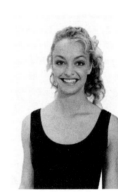

Gina Simontacchi

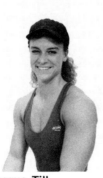

Jacque Till

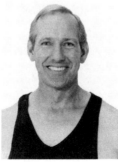

Ken Sprague

Get fit with the best names in physical fitness and strength training.

These books are available at your bookstore or wherever books are sold, or, for your convenience, we'll send them directly to you. Call 1-800-631-8571 (press 1 for inquiries and orders) or fill out the coupon below and send it to:

The Berkley Publishing Group
390 Murray Hill Parkway, Department B
East Rutherford, NJ 07073

	ISBN	U.S.	CAN
____ *Sports Strength* by Ken Sprague	399-51802-9	$16.95	$22.50
____ *The Gold's Gym Book of Weight Training* by Ken Sprague	399-51846-0	$14.00	$18.50
____ *Weight and Strength Training for Kids and Teenagers* by Ken Sprague	874-77643-0	$12.95	
____ *Gold's Gym Book of Strength Training* by Ken Sprague	399-51863-0	$14.00	$18.50
____ *High-Performance Bodybuilding* by John Parrillo and Maggie Greenwood-Robinson	399-51771-5	$16.00	$21.00
____ *Big* by Ellington Darden, Ph.D.	399-51630-1	$16.00	$21.00
____ *Bigger Muscles in 42 Days* by Ellington Darden, Ph.D.	399-51706-5	$16.00	$21.00
____ *High-Intensity Strength Training* by Ellington Darden, Ph.D.	399-51770-7	$16.00	$21.00
____ *Massive Muscles in 10 Weeks* by Ellington Darden, Ph.D.	399-51340-X	$16.00	$21.00
____ *New High-Intensity Bodybuilding* by Ellington Darden, Ph.D.	399-51614-X	$15.95	$20.95
____ *The Six-Week Fat-to-Muscle Makeover* by Ellington Darden, Ph.D.	399-51562-3	$9.95	$12.95
____ *High-Intensity Home Training* by Ellington Darden, Ph.D.	399-51840-1	$15.95	$20.95
____ *John Parrillo's 50 Workout Secrets* by John Parrillo and Maggie Greenwood-Robinson (Available July 1994)	399-51862-2	$16.00	$21.00

Subtotal $ _____

Postage & handling* $ _____

Sales tax (CA, NY, NJ, PA) $ _____

Total amount due $ _____

Payable in U.S. funds (no cash orders accepted).
$15.00 minimum for credit card orders.

*Postage & handling: $2.50 for 1 book, 75¢ each additional book up to a maximum of $6.25.

Enclosed is my ☐ check ☐ money order
Please charge my ☐ Visa ☐ Mastercard ☐ American Express

Card #_____ Expiration date _____

Signature as on charge card _____

Name _____

Address _____

City _____ State _____ Zip _____

Please allow six weeks for delivery. Prices subject to change without notice.